The

Alpha
Solution

For Permanent Weight Loss

The Alpha Solution

For Permanent Weight Loss

Harness the Power of Your Subconscious Mind to
Change Your Relationship with Food—Forever

Ronald J. Glassman, Ph.D., M.P.H.

with Mollie Doyle

Broadway Books
New York

PUBLISHED BY BROADWAY BOOKS

Published in the United States by Broadway Books, an imprint of The Doubleday Broadway Publishing Group, a division of Random House, Inc., New York.

www.broadwaybooks.com

Book design by rlf design

Library of Congress Cataloging-in-Publication Data
Glassman, Ronald J.
The Alpha solution for permanent weight loss : harness the power of your subconscious mind to change your relationship with food—forever / Ronald J. Glassman with Mollie Doyle. — 1st ed.
p. cm.
1. Weight loss. 2. Hypnotism—Therapeutic use. 3. Neurolinguistic programming. I. Doyle, Mollie. II. Title.
RM222.2.G538 2007
615.8'512—dc22
2006034648

ISBN: 978-0-7679-2591-4

PRINTED IN THE UNITED STATES OF AMERICA

10 9 8 7 6 5 4 3 2 1

First Edition

In Honor

This book is dedicated to Meryl,
my wife and best friend.

I also dedicate this book to every
person who has ever struggled
with their weight.

In Memory

Moe "Doc" Leff
Stuart M. Corsover
Alma Berkowitz Corsover Goldberg

The brain is the only programmable organ in the body.

Choose the direction you want to program yours . . .

and enjoy the journey.

—Ron Glassman

Contents

Acknowledgments

I could not have made my way to this place without the following individuals and institutions providing inspiration and support through the journey. Words to express my heartfelt appreciation don't yet exist.

Dr. Albert Einstein; Rutgers, Columbia, and Harvard Universities; Dr. Milton Erickson, the father of medical hypnosis and neurolinguistic programming; Dr. Jeffrey Schwartz; Dr. Daniel Amen; Dr. Herbert Spiegel; Dr. David Spiegel; Dr. Ben Carson; Dr. Herbert Benson of the Harvard Medical School Mind-Body Institute; Dr. Joy Hirsch of Columbia University College of Physicians and Surgeons; Dr. Jack Elinson of Columbia University School of Public Health; Dr. Dave Thomas and Dr. Sherry Gorelick of Rutgers University; Dr. Zita Norwalk Polsky; Dr. J. Paul Teusink; and Dr. Jamie Feldman.

Special appreciation goes to Meryl, who inspires me daily; Mollie Doyle, the best writer of all; and Brian DeFiore, the greatest literary agent of all. I also sincerely thank K.K., who referred A.T., who referred R.L., the person who said to me, "You know, Ron, you really should write a book" and ultimately got Brian and me in the same room. I also thank everyone at Random House Publishing, especially Ann Campbell, my extraordinary editor, and her always-on-top-of-things assistant, Laura Lee Mattingly.

And finally, my wonderful office support staff in the New Jersey and Manhattan offices, without whom I would not know whether I was coming or going!

The
Alpha
Solution

For Permanent Weight Loss

Thin Is a
State of Mind

Chapter One

Even when I was little, I was big.

—William "Refrigerator" Perry,

Chicago Bears defensive tackle, on his weight,

quoted in *Life*, January 1986

Fat is not our destiny or our destination, but for many of us it feels like it is. I should know. I was 75 pounds overweight and struggled with food for the first twenty years of my life. It was an endless and losing battle of trying to gain control over what I was eating and how I was eating it. I now know that I was not alone. Nor are you. According to the Centers for Disease Control's National Center for Health Statistics, more than 66 percent of Americans are overweight. And about half of this group have graduated to qualify as obese.[1] In 2005, 112,000 people died due to a poor diet and inactivity.[2] In fact, being overweight or obese is the second leading cause of preventable death in the United States.[3] And more than 50 percent of U.S. adults did not engage in physical activity at the minimum recommended level.[4]

These are big numbers, but nothing like the whopping $30 billion the American Obesity Association reports that we Americans annually spend on weight reduction products, services, and programs to try to get help.[5] Clearly, the struggle to gain control over our expanding waist-lines is huge—economically, mentally, physically, even spiritually.

To make matters worse, gaining weight is incredibly easy. Just add a Starbucks Venti Caffè Mocha Espresso, which is 290 calories (with low-fat milk and no whipped cream), to your daily intake for twelve days and you can gain a pound.[6] But burning the necessary 3,500 calo-ries to lose this pound is hard work. The average person would have to rigorously walk for twelve and a half hours to burn these twelve mochas off.

And, as you know, there are tens of thousands of diet books, pro-grams, philosophies, tapes, and camps that promise to help people lose weight. But, as you also know, these programs and books rarely, if ever, work to achieve healthy, safe, and long-term weight loss. In fact, hun-dreds of studies by venerable institutions such as the Federal Trade Commission, the Food and Drug Administration, and the National Association of Attorneys General have shown that 95 percent of peo-ple who use weight-loss programs—from books and tapes to medical approaches—with some success can't keep the weight off for more than a year. And the 95 percent who gain the weight back, more often than not, gain back more than they lost.[7] The truth is, not one single diet, diet book, diet program, diet tape, or diet camp does for the over-weight person what he or she really needs to do: *establish a different relationship with food.*

Why don't these programs work? Because they deal only with the food we're eating, not the person eating the food. They don't address the hardwired psychological desire to overeat, the cravings for "feel-good" foods, or the urge to snack when there's no real need for actual sustenance. If eating were just a biological matter of fueling our bodies the way we fuel up our cars, we'd all be thin. But for most of us, eating to supply our bodies with energy is secondary.

- Eating is a cultural event. We go out to eat, seeking new and unusual experiences.

- Eating is social. It's an arena where we relate to others and they relate to us.

- Eating is psychological. It's a way for us to relax, soothe, and reward ourselves for a job well done or another day survived.

- Eating is pleasurable. It's an instant jolt to the brain's pleasure center, which for many of us is powerful, bordering on addictive.

As a result, many of us wind up eating more than we need to, and we gain weight. Then we try to lose it. If we do lose it, most of us gain the weight back. And then we try to lose the weight again. . . . This psychological relationship with food choreographs an endless and tortured dance in which food is our friend, then our enemy, then our friend, and on it goes. According to the American Obesity Association, 40 percent of American women and 25 percent of American men are actively trying to lose weight at any given time.[8]

The Solution to Our Weight Problems Lies in Our Minds

As a visiting scientist and guest lecturer at Columbia University Medical School's Center for Neurobiology and Behavior, I have the unique opportunity to view the working human brain as it thinks. After studying thousands of brains and the way they process thoughts, I can say with confidence that the answer to the struggle with food and weight lies between our ears. The answer to our fat problem? Rewire our brains. We get fat because our minds think fat.

In our evolved society of social and psychological eating, our subconscious mind has been conditioned (like any muscle or organ in our body) to tell us to eat more than we need to. **Our brains have been supersized.** So we overeat, crave foods, and snack unnecessarily. And if our subconscious mind has been trained for this behavior, no matter what diet or exercise regime we embrace, the subconscious mind will always override our conscious, logical desire to be thin.

The only way to break any habit is to have both the conscious and subconscious minds agree to do things differently. Until our conscious desire is reflected by the subconscious mind, our two minds will remain in conflict and the habit will remain unbroken. But when the conscious and subconscious minds agree, the conscious desire becomes subconscious action. There is no conflict and no ambivalence. What we think we want to do becomes what we actually do more easily.

This is why using talk therapy alone to address issues such as overeating or smoking rarely works. While talk therapy is extremely valuable, helping the client to consciously understand why he or she has a habit and that the habit may be hurtful, it rarely speaks to or changes the subconscious mind. The conscious and subconscious minds remain in conflict and the habit remains unbroken. The key, therefore, to changing any unwanted habit—from nail biting to overeating—is to rewire the subconscious mind to agree with the conscious mind's desire. Both sides of our head have to be on the same page.

After generations of research, study, and experience, many scientists, doctors, and therapists agree that medical hypnosis is the most effective and permanent method for helping their clients reframe the unhealthy habits and behaviors that are wired in their subconscious mind. An astounding 96 percent of my clients have successfully used medical hypnosis and changed their subconscious mind's unhealthy picture of food to mirror their conscious mind's image of healthy eating and lost weight—without restrictions, often without exercise, and without the struggle and deprivation associated with dieting.*

The Alpha Solution

Contrary to popular understanding, hypnosis or trance is a naturally occurring state. Scientists call it the alpha state, where our brains cycle at a rate of 8–14 times per second, which is slower than our normal functioning rate, but faster than the sleep rate. Daydreaming, the tranquil feeling we have just before and as we fall asleep, meditation, or being mesmerized by a movie or a long stretch of highway are all exam-

---

* This 96 percent success rate is based on a survey of 25 percent of my clients from every walk of life. Scientists cannot follow up on every (total population) subject. Therefore, the 25 percent sample is a representative group from the total population and attempts to replicate demographically the entire population (a cross-section of males, females, ages, races, education levels, etc.). This is standard scientific methodology.

ples of natural hypnotic states where our brain has slowed down and we feel completely at ease and very relaxed. We feel good in this state because our body's stress hormones are significantly lower.

Scientists have proven the healing powers of this alpha state. Because of the decrease in stress hormones, the alpha state facilitates the body's ability to lower its blood pressure and blood sugar levels. So for more than fifty years doctors and scientists have been capitalizing upon the alpha state's natural healing abilities, using meditation and medical hypnosis to treat high blood pressure and diabetes. And because of the increased endorphin levels that often accompany this state, scientists and doctors have also used medical hypnosis or meditation to treat depression, anxiety, pain, and chronic diseases such as heart conditions, high blood pressure, and the side effects that accompany AIDS and cancer. Some of the most compelling evidence of the power of the mind and its role in health and healing has been found by researchers at the Harvard Medical School Mind-Body Institute, where I do ongoing postdoctoral training.

In 1971, expanding on the work of Swiss Nobel laureate Dr. Walter R. Hess, Dr. Herbert Benson and his colleagues at Harvard documented the opposite of the fight-or-flight (stress) response. They called it the Relaxation Response. The Relaxation Response is induced by focusing on the breath. They say, "This results in decreased metabolism, heart rate, blood pressure, and rate of breathing, as well as slower brain waves."[9] Sounds good, doesn't it? Well, it gets even better. The Relaxation Response has also been shown to increase fertility, appease chronic pain, and strengthen the ability to cope with stress.[10]

But beyond using the alpha state to address and treat our physical ailments, scientists, doctors, and therapists also induce the alpha state using medical hypnosis to treat unhealthy subconscious thought patterning—from attention deficit disorder and obsessive-compulsive disorder to overeating. The alpha state is like a corridor between our conscious and unconscious minds. At the end of this hallway is the door to the subconscious. And, as you know, when we have access to something, we can talk to it and change it. In other words, unlike any other state in the human experience, the alpha state provides us with the opportunity to change our subconscious thought patterns. This means we can use medical hypnosis to change any unwanted behaviors—from performance anxiety to overeating. In fact, using magnetic resonance imaging (MRI), scientists see a difference in a person's brain after just minutes of experiencing the meditative/hypnotic state.

While our feelings about food may be complicated, the process of changing our fundamental food habits using medical hypnosis is not.

Because all hypnosis is self-hypnosis, when clients come to see me, I tell them that I am not going to do something *to* them. I am not a magician. I cannot make anyone change or control anyone's mind. The only person I can change or control is myself, and this goes for everyone. As a medical hypnosis practitioner, I am essentially a trainer. I train people how to use their minds in an empowering way. I teach people how to induce the alpha state and use suggestion to change their unhealthy subconscious thought patterns. I am constantly telling my clients that the work we do in my office is almost irrelevant to their healing process. The healing comes from their use of the tool of hypnosis to change the environment in their minds. This is why I can talk to someone on the phone and teach that person how to use medical hypnosis even if he or she is halfway around the world. This is why I can teach someone how to use medical hypnosis for weight loss and control in a book.

For the last twenty-five years, I have used medical hypnosis to help thousands of people—from barely educated to overeducated, from financially struggling to wealthy, from Arizona to New Zealand—change their subconscious minds and lose weight. Medical hypnosis has facilitated my clients' conscious desire to be thin, fit, and healthy by drawing a new "food blueprint" in their subconscious mind to reflect their conscious picture of healthy eating. I have found that this method permanently changes a person's relationship with food so that the problem foods and behaviors—from chocolate to binging—are either erased or modified. My clients no longer have the conscious/subconscious conflict that prevents them from losing weight. With medical hypnosis they change the "fat thinking" to "thin thinking" and the weight comes off.

For example, one of Hollywood's most powerful producers came to see me a few years ago. She was 50 pounds overweight. As you know, being even 5 pounds overweight in Hollywood is a sin. But what was even worse was that her husband had started to make jokes about her weight. When this happened, she was devastated. Even her home had become a hostile environment, a place of humiliation.

Fortunately, after spending thousands of dollars on diet programs, fat farms, and low-carb food delivery services with no success, she heard about another approach: medical hypnosis. Two of her aunts and her grandfather had been to see me. All of them had changed their relationship with food and had lost the weight they wanted to lose. She got my number from one of her aunts, called my office, made an appointment, bought a plane ticket, and flew across the country to see me the following month.

On her first visit, we talked about her life. She told me that she usually had three or four TV shows and movies in production at any given time. And when she wasn't hanging out on freezing sets in the middle of Alaska, eating and drinking to keep warm and calm her nerves, she was in LA having breakfast, lunch, and dinner with agents, producers, directors, and actors. She told me that some days, she felt like she was going from plate to plate.

She also told me that the craft trucks on the sets were her own personal hell. She could not resist the high-carbohydrate, high-fat, high-sugar foods—danishes, donuts, mochas, pizza, pasta, macaroni and cheese, chocolates—that were perpetually on display and available for the working crews. Just thinking about a craft truck made her hungry.

We did two medical hypnosis sessions in the space of a week where I taught her how to use the alpha state to draw a new food blueprint in her mind. In the year that followed, the producer lost 45 pounds. Four years later, she is now 55 pounds thinner and fit, has no struggle with food, can walk by a craft truck and feel nothing, and—most importantly—does not use food to manage her stress levels, a behavior that was actually creating more stress!

Throughout this book, you will hear dozens of success stories like this one: The woman who gained her college freshman 40 because of a serious peanut butter habit and used medical hypnosis and lost the weight. The high-finance banker who ate his way through stressful deals and lost 100 pounds with the help of medical hypnosis. A mother who couldn't get a grip on snacking to lose 10 post-pregnancy pounds and finally did with medical hypnosis. The psychiatrist who had tried everything from Atkins to analysis to kick his four-bagel-a-day habit and finally tried medical hypnosis and lost 60 pounds. They are just like you, and you can be just like them if you let the Alpha Solution work for you.

I Practice What I Preach

Beyond helping thousands of people end lifelong painful battles with food, I also know the power of medical hypnosis from personal experience.

I was an obese child and adolescent who tried every available diet and exercise program. By the time I was a sophomore in college, I was 75 pounds overweight and lived in a constant fight with food. I wondered, "How did I get this way? Why is food such a struggle for me? Why is it so hard for me to turn any morsel down? Why is it that I can do everything else so well—get good grades, be popular, have great friends and girlfriends, be a good son—yet cannot control myself when it comes to eating?" I was nineteen, and no matter what I did, my mind continued to call for me to eat pizzas, mashed potatoes, and junk food. I also binged on high-carb foods several times a week, including secret binges in the middle of the night. (One-third of overeaters engage in nocturnal binging.)

I was and am intimately familiar with the conscious/subconscious conflict and the overriding power of the subconscious mind. How did this battle in my mind arise? At a very young age, my brain was trained to be fat—to use food as a tool for soothing emotional upset and alleviating stress.

I was raised in a home with complicated messages about food. My father taught me to believe that being fat was desirable. He had grown up in the heart of the Ukraine during one of the most harrowing famines in all of history: the Black Famine, in which seven million people died of starvation. Fortunately, my father survived, but not without the harrowing memory of watching friends and family go hungry and ultimately lose their lives. So when he had a son in America, the land of plenty, he wanted me to be well fed. A plump child to him was the sign of success and good fortune. In his family, the phrase "You're looking thin" was the ultimate condemnation. So he encouraged me to clean my plate, eat large portions, and be heavy.

As a registered nurse, my mother knew that obesity was not healthy for a child, and she encouraged me to eat lean protein and vegetables. But, due to her schedule, she was often absent during the afternoon or for evening meals. So I was mainly under my father's influence. My afternoons and evenings became focused on hanging out and eating.

And then, at eleven o'clock at night, my mother would come home from the three-to-eleven shift. She would be exhausted and starving from yet another stressful day at the hospital and would come say hi before going into the kitchen to eat. More often than not, I would get up and follow her there. She'd usually eat her dinner and then we would have ice cream and cookies or cake. This was our way of bonding and her reward to herself after a long, hard day's work. But eating late at night and then going to bed almost guarantees weight gain. Your body has no time to use the calories you've ingested, so instead it stores them as fat. I learned from my mother that food was a bonding, soothing, stress-relieving reward for having survived another day. This habit of getting up to eat after going to bed is also what jump-started my nocturnal binging behavior. And with all of these messages encouraging me to eat—clean my plate, eat to bond, eat to relieve stress, eat in the middle of the night—you can see why I began to use food as something other than fuel for my mind and body.

I ate Twinkies, potato chips, pretzels, and french fries in large volumes. A box of Dunkin' Donuts. An entire pizza. Two plates of mashed potatoes. A pint of ice cream. And guess what? The pounds settled in and stuck.

When I was twelve, I went on my first diet. An extraordinary teacher took interest in my struggle with food and helped me to lose 50 pounds. I did this by limiting my carbohydrate intake to 50 grams per day and eating mostly protein. I felt great, met my first love, Lori, and thought I would never look back. But despite all of my newfound happiness, my programmed subconscious desire to overeat overpowered my conscious desire to be thin, and I found myself obsessed with food and eating all over again. Within a year, I was 40 pounds overweight.

As a teenager, I was overwhelmed and shocked by my powerlessness over food and my desire to eat. I read nutrition books and diet books and even joined a Weight Watchers program with my mother, which was humiliating because I was not just the only male in the group but also the only person under forty! We had to weigh in at the front of the room. If you lost weight, everyone clapped. If you gained, you could hear a pin drop. I did this for a couple of months and lost about 20 pounds. But then one day I missed what I wasn't eating and took a bite out of a Suzi Q, and there was no looking back. I ate a container of vanilla frosting, several packages of Suzi Qs, and a canned milkshake. And my cravings came surging back with the force of a rocket. Every day, I would stockpile crap in the attic; later I would sneak upstairs and snack. Clearly, none of this reading or talking about dieting had helped me, as I continued to gain weight.

By then, it was the late seventies, the era of marathons, aerobics, and gyms, and I began to believe that my weight problem was due to the fact that I had not found the right form of exercise. So I started lifting weights. Once again, I lost 50 pounds. I competed in amateur power-lifting competitions, was nationally ranked, and was once again praised by my teachers and peers for losing weight. But then I hurt my back and the call of food and excess weight returned.

As time went on, I rationalized the decision to give up on trying to control my eating and be thin by focusing on my other successes: I was an honors student at a much-lauded university, I was popular, and I was going out with, in my opinion, one of the most brilliant and beautiful women on campus. So with all of this, why did I need to be thin? Other than better health and a potentially longer life, what would being thin get me?

Fortunately, that year in a psychology class I stumbled upon the work of Dr. Milton Erickson, a physician, psychiatrist, and psychotherapist who has been called "the most creative, perceptive, and ingenious psychotherapeutic master of all time."[11] Practicing in the mid-twentieth century, Dr. Erickson was the first person to explore the powers of neurolinguistic programming and neurolinguistic psychology, and is the father of medical hypnosis.

In his work, Dr. Erickson defines medical hypnosis as "communication" and as "concentrating *exclusively* on your own thoughts, values, memories and beliefs about life." In his writings, he also describes the trance state as "active unconscious learning."[12]

Intrigued by Dr. Erickson's work, I did more research and found that, contrary to my belief that hypnosis was just a magician's parlor trick, medical hypnosis had been recognized and used by members of the American Medical Association for fifty years to treat pain, to control the nausea associated with cancer treatment, and to manage anxiety. Most importantly, it had been phenomenally successful with habit and behavior modification. Perhaps most enlightening was the fact that hypnosis had been used for a couple of hundred years as an effective pain reduction tool.

I wondered if medical hypnosis had been used to help people modify their relationships with food. After class, I asked my psychology professor, Dr. Dave Thomas, if he thought that medical hypnosis would help me with my weight problem. Dr. Thomas said that it had been used for food and weight issues and might indeed help me. He suggested that I go to the school's student health center and ask if anyone was trained in Ericksonian hypnosis. Feeling hopeful (once again) about the prospect of something really helping me with my weight, I left class and went straight to the student health center, where to my surprise I found not just one but two Ericksonian-trained therapists. I made an appointment.

During my first appointment, the therapist explained to me that all hypnosis is self-hypnosis, that I would be in total control, and that I would just feel more relaxed than usual. I learned that, as we've seen, a trance state is a natural state called the alpha state. More importantly, I learned that when people are in the alpha state, they can become highly focused on their internal reality and subconscious mind. The therapist explained that this ability to focus on the nonconscious thought is why medical hypnosis is the best tool for behavior modification and reframing—it is essentially talk therapy for the subconscious mind, allowing us to suggest the changes we consciously desire. In my case, I could talk to my subconscious mind and change the unhealthy messages and food patterns into a pattern for healthy eating.

I then talked to the therapist about my fraught relationship with food—that I felt like a servant to the overbearing master: cravings. I also talked about what I wanted my relationship with food to be—that I would enjoy food, but it wouldn't have a hold on me. Then the therapist taught me how to use self-hypnosis, providing me with a customized audio script that reflected the relationship with food I envisioned: that I would be in control of food and want to make healthier choices. He also told me that in order to lose weight, I should listen to this customized recording as I fell asleep every night for several weeks. This repetition would enforce the new relationship I imagined. I could not fully believe that hypnosis and neurolinguistic programming would really help me to achieve my lifelong aspiration to eat in a healthy way, but I decided to give it a try. After all, what did I have to lose?

Well, it turned out that I had weight to lose. Within days, I immediately felt a difference in some aspects of my relationship with food. My unhealthy eating habits had abated, and I was making better choices—salad instead of two dinner rolls with butter, smaller portions, steamed foods instead of fried. And, amazingly, after the first hypnosis session, my nocturnal binging stopped completely! Twenty minutes of rewiring and this lifelong, devastating behavior was over! The nine foods I had identified as my particular triggers—bread, pasta, peanut butter, chocolate, cake, cookies, pizza, mashed potatoes, and French toast—also had less draw, and I turned to them less. I didn't need to eat a second meal of ice cream and cookies at ten o'clock while studying. Potato chips and pretzels didn't sing to me while I was reading. Within a month, there was a nearly 100 percent change in my relationship with food. The pendulum had swung from the worst possible eating behavior to eating the way a thin, healthy athlete would. But I wasn't dieting. I didn't feel deprived. I had simply experienced a change of mind.

Within a year, I lost more than 50 pounds. And twenty-five years later, I am 100 pounds lighter. I am thin and fit, and most importantly, I have never struggled with food since the medical hypnosis treatment permanently rewired my subconscious overeating mind to be a healthy-eating mind. I eat like a thin person. To ensure that I will never struggle with food again, every few weeks I listen to the recording of my second session with the therapist. This replenishes and reinforces my brain's healthy food blueprint. To combat stress—the number-one relapse trigger for overeaters—I also meditate for twenty minutes nearly every day. Meditation is a wonderful stress reliever and also helps me see my subconscious thoughts, which puts me in further control of my choices and actions. I can see when my mind is wandering to food and address it objectively. This produces a sense of empowerment—*not* deprivation!

The reason why medical hypnosis succeeded when everything else failed is that it spoke to my subconscious mind directly, rewiring it to agree with my conscious desire to change my relationship with food. And once my subconscious brain was "reset" to agree with my conscious desire to be thin, I lost weight. Easily.

This life-changing experience led me to pursue a degree in public health and social sciences and to spend the last twenty-five years working in health care—specifically with medical hypnosis. Aside from my convincing personal experience, my choice to specialize in medical hypnosis was further inspired by my graduate studies in public health at Columbia. Public health is essentially the study of disease prevention. And, based upon my research, medical hypnosis was the most effective method—for some things far better than pharmaceuticals—that I found to help prevent disease, from lowering high blood pressure to addressing other stress-related disorders such as inflammatory bowel syndrome. In a way, medical hypnosis is the penicillin of approaches in that it can enhance the treatment of a profoundly diverse group of complaints. But unlike penicillin, which is an outside resource, medical hypnosis uses a person's own strength—imagination, creativity, and physiology—to change and heal.

Since then, my personal experience working with thousands of clients and my studies at Columbia University Medical School's Center for Neurobiology and Behavior have afforded me the opportunity to become one of this country's foremost experts in medical hypnosis. In fact, I was recently named "Researcher of the Year" by the International Association of Counselors and Therapists.

You Don't Need a Degree to Do It

As an expert in medical hypnosis and based on my own personal experience, I know that you don't need to have a Ph.D., be a medical doctor, or even be a therapist to put the natural hypnotic state to work. *Everyone* can learn how to use medical hypnosis and attain his or her ideal relationship with food and a slim and healthy body. Moreover, whether you know it or not, you are already an expert on your struggle with food. You know most of your triggers and what your "gotta have it" foods are. These two pieces of information are all you need to use your natural alpha state to modify your food preferences.

A wealthy Connecticut housewife in her early sixties recently called me in a panic. She was just 5 pounds overweight, but she told me that these few pounds were her torture. She had fought these same pounds for nearly forty years, and even though she was a size two, she felt better when she was 5 pounds thinner. She was willing to do anything— chant, have a séance, pray, pay me millions—if I could help her lose the weight.

Knowing that a struggle with food and weight is a struggle no matter how much weight you're battling, I began asking her about her background and what her relationship to food was like.

She told me that she exercised and that she didn't binge, overeat, purge, snack, or have cravings, but she was diabetic and had high blood pressure. I was about to tell her I was stumped when she said, "Well, I do have one food habit, but it's just a fruit."

"What fruit?" I asked.

"Watermelon."

My Sherlock Holmes brain went, "Aha!" While low in fat, watermelon is very high in sugar. Just ten cubes of watermelon have 7.6 grams of sugar, which is almost as much sugar as a Hershey's chocolate bar.[13] The woman told me that she was obsessed with watermelon, that she would eat two cups of it four to five times a day. She didn't like to drink water, so she ate watermelon to hydrate herself. I knew right away that this seemingly innocuous habit was behind those 5 pounds. When the body is overloaded with sugar—from too much fruit or too much soda—it turns the extra sugar into fat. I also knew that the watermelon was contributing to her diabetes. This amount of sugar would be an assault on any body, throwing insulin levels off balance.

Even though I knew I had the answer to her 5-pound problem and diabetes, I was curious about her high blood pressure, so I continued asking her what else she was eating. Did she cook? Go out? She told me that she didn't eat out much, but didn't really cook either. She would just pop a Lean Cuisine meal into her microwave. Another "Aha!" While low in calories, frozen foods like Lean Cuisine are loaded with salt. For instance, the Chicken Tuscan has 780 milligrams of salt per serving.[14] I told her to go to her freezer and look at the sodium levels on one of the Lean Cuisine boxes. When she read them, she gasped, "I had no idea. No wonder my blood pressure is so high."

I told her that I could help her, and suggested she come see me. She refused for a myriad of reasons—she didn't want to make the drive, didn't want to be seen entering my office, and didn't want to have to explain what she was doing to her husband. So I taught her how to use medical hypnosis over the phone.

I talked to her for about an hour and a half, showing her how to use medical hypnosis and neurolinguistic programming, which we will talk about in Chapter 4, to control her cravings for watermelon and Lean Cuisine. I told her that if she needed to eat fruit, she should eat strawberries, which are very low in sugar but would pack the same refreshing experience as watermelon cubes.

She called about a month and a half later to tell me that not only had she lost the 5 pounds, but her blood sugar levels had dropped from 130 to 90 and she was off her blood pressure medication. She also told me that she felt liberated. She estimated that before our phone conversation she had spent at least three hours a day thinking about food. Now she had a lot more time for her family—especially her grandchildren.

Watermelon, frozen meals, fattening cuisine, dark chocolate, milk chocolate, chocolate milk, fast food, slow food, 800 pounds, 10 pounds, unwanted postpregnancy weight, car eaters, drive-through, afternoon snackers, attic storers, a person who could not drive by New York City's Second Avenue Deli without ordering a corned beef and pastrami sandwich, bulimics, addicts, exercise fanatics . . . I have seen it all. And I have helped 96 percent of those people permanently change their subconscious relationship with food and lose weight. Without a struggle. Forever.

The next eleven chapters of this book are designed to replicate the *exact* process that clients go through when they come to see me, and allow you to do it for yourself. The only requirement for you to be successful with the Alpha Solution is to have a true desire to revolutionize your relationship with food and a willingness to change your mind.

This willingness is the key, since all hypnosis is self-hypnosis. No one—no doctor, therapist, spouse, or child—can do it for you. If you want a new relationship with food, you, and only you, must be willing to embrace this process, answering the questions I will ask you honestly, following my instructions rigorously, and listening religiously to the tape or CD you'll make.

If you are feeling excited about this process, then you are almost ready to move on to Chapter 2. But before you move ahead, I have an assignment for you.

The Life Log

As you read this book and follow my prescription for safe and permanent weight loss, I want you to keep a Life Log. In this Life Log, I want you to record the following:

The date, including the day of the week

What you woke up feeling like—happy, sad, depressed, anxious, late, frustrated, overwhelmed (this entry can be one word or an entire page)

What you ate for breakfast, including where you ate it, how you ate it, and who was around

How you felt after breakfast—full, satisfied, hungry, guilty

What you ate midmorning or when you got to work or while you worked or drove around, including where you ate it, how you ate it, and who was around

How you felt after this snack—full, satisfied, hungry, guilty

What you ate for lunch, including where you ate it, how you ate it, and who was around

How you felt after lunch—full, satisfied, hungry, guilty

What you ate for a midafternoon snack or all afternoon, including where you ate it, how you ate it, and who was around

How you felt after this snack—full, satisfied, hungry, guilty

What you ate when you got home, including where you ate it, how you ate it, and who was around

How you felt after this snack—full, satisfied, hungry, guilty

What you ate for dinner, including where you ate it, how you ate it, and who was around

How you felt after dinner—full, satisfied, hungry, guilty

What you ate after dinner (while watching TV, hanging out, at the movies, etc.), including where you ate it, how you ate it, and who was around

How you felt after this snack—full, satisfied, hungry, guilty

What you ate before going to bed or in the middle of the night, including where you ate it, how you ate it, and who was around

How you felt after this snack—full, satisfied, hungry, guilty

What you went to bed feeling like—happy, sad, depressed, anxious, late, frustrated, overwhelmed (again, this entry can be one word or an entire page)

Significant events or stresses that may have happened over the course of your day—your kid stained your new carpet, the boss overlooked you for an assignment, your spouse or partner behaved inconsiderately, there was a ton of traffic on the way home, they didn't have your favorite brand of shampoo at the market

Don't worry, I am not going to have you counting calories in the next chapter! Nor am I going to have you read this out loud to someone or perform some ridiculous ritual where you eventually burn the journal along with five white horsehairs and some incense. The Life Log is not about shame or humiliation. Nor is it just about food. It is about *you*—your life, how you move through it, and most importantly, how you feel day to day, as most overeaters, snackers, and bingers eat for emotional reasons. The Life Log is about awareness and knowledge, which is the essence of medical hypnosis. Medical hypnosis is about becoming aware of who we are and how we respond to the outside world, then reshaping our knee-jerk reactions to the people, places, and things in our lives so that we respond in a way that is nurturing, satisfying, and healthy for us.

Sure, you may know the broad strokes of your struggle with food, but recording the fight day after day will give you a much more detailed and accurate picture of what needs to be reshaped—so that your reaction to your boss yelling at you is no longer eating half a box of donuts (or even one), but a five-minute meditation or a walk around the block to clear your head.

As for the notebook, don't make a big deal out of what kind of notebook it should be. Just go to the drugstore and buy something that immediately speaks to you and can easily be carried around.

Do you need to keep a Life Log to use medical hypnosis to gain control over your struggle with food? No.

That said, a resistance to following this part of the process does suggest that you may have some ambivalence about *really* wanting to lose weight. It may be that you've already done four different logs on four different diet programs and just aren't convinced that it's time well spent. But I encourage you to make an effort to participate in this part of the process, as it can also be a great source of positive reinforcement. As you get deeper into the process of using medical hypnosis, you will have a concrete record that shows the dramatic difference between a life locked in struggle with food and a life that is free.

And now, if you are ready to begin your liberation, turn the page.

The Solution Is Not in the Refrigerator— It's Within You

Chapter Two

Your brain is the hardware of your soul.

—Dr. Daniel G. Amen

Medical hypnosis is about forging a new path for yourself. In contrast to other diet programs, it's not about making outside changes—trying a new exercise or taking food out of your cabinets or never eating in a restaurant again (though you will probably be less inclined to seek gourmet dining experiences and more inclined to stock your fridge with healthier foods such as fruits and lean proteins). The Alpha Solution for Permanent Weight Loss capitalizes upon your brain's natural ability to picture, learn, and establish new behaviors. You were not born with a preference for fries and pizza; your brain was *trained* to crave these things.

Medical Hypnosis Is an Inside Job

As you will learn in Chapters 3 and 4, medical hypnosis uses our imagination and words to rewire our subconscious minds, redrawing our minds to create patterns of healthy eating. This redrawing takes determination, work, and time; it is not magic. Using medical hypnosis to rewire your brain for healthy eating takes a commitment—to yourself and to your life.

If your experience is anything like mine, you've probably heard the C-word (that's *commitment*) from every diet program, book, CD, and tape. And you probably don't want to hear another definition of commitment or about how making a commitment will change your life. You just want a solution. I understand. So we won't spend a ton of time on this, but it is also no accident that every program talks about commitment. There is real value in making a firm resolution to try your best, to do something thoroughly. But unlike these other programs, medical hypnosis is not about dieting or deprivation. It is about changing your mind to change your life. If you are honest with yourself, follow the directions in this book, and are diligent about listening to the CD you will be recording, you will see dramatic changes in your life before you know it.

Are you prepared for change?

Can you imagine yourself not in a struggle with food? Can you see yourself looking and feeling lean, strong, and healthy? When I was in college and had fallen off the diet wagon again, I got to the point where I thought, "This is it. I am meant to be fat. I am meant to eat. There is nothing I can do. I am okay with being obese for the rest of my life. It's okay that I feel awful—tired, embarrassed, ashamed. It's okay that I will probably die sooner. I don't care. I give up." I just could not envision a life where I was not locked in a constant struggle with food, or where I was not dieting and feeling deprived.

But the truth is that a part of me was also scared to be thin and free of the struggle. Although I had been thin before, the struggle never ceased. My entire life was oriented around my fight with food: buying it, hiding it, ordering it, eating it, buying more, binging, feeling ashamed, trying to eat less, forcing myself to exercise. I could not imagine what would happen if I lost the weight. It was a huge part of my identity, and it had always served as an excuse to remain passive rather than reaching out to achieve my full potential.

So maybe you're like me and the idea of change is really scary. Maybe you think the known is easier than the unknown. Being in a struggle with food makes life predictable: You know you will spend the bulk of your time eating and thinking about eating or not eating. On the other hand, becoming lean, strong, and healthy might mean change—something unpredictable could happen. Living in the unknown is hard, but in my experience, after trying both, I can say that it is filled with infinitely more pleasure and joy—way more than any food or binge ever brought me. Do you think stashing away food in my attic was joyful? That binging on it in the middle of the night was empowering? Even though it was predictable, it tore me apart.

For years, remaining obese allowed me to not claim my life or be a responsible adult. As an out-of-control eater, I was not responsible. Food was in control, not me. So when I finally took the action of redrawing my brain's pattern for food, I was also saying, "I control food. Food cannot control me." For the first time in my life, I was in charge. I became the adult. It was challenging, terrifying—and exhilarating.

Let me tell you a story about another person who was scared to lose weight. A few years ago a client named John came to see me. He was a phenomenally successful fifty-three-year-old financial consultant who was a smoker and was also 100 pounds overweight. As with all my clients, in the first session I asked John about his stress level. I learned that he was crumbling under pressure. At home, he had two children, one of whom had Asperger's syndrome. To complicate the home life picture, he and his wife were having a hard time. At work, he had to make cold calls to potential clients for four hours each day to make enough money to support the luxurious lifestyle his family had become accustomed to. John was trying to relieve his stress by smoking and eating, which, ironically, add more stress to the body.

I asked him what bad habit he wanted to address first. He told me he wanted to stop smoking first, as it drove his wife nuts and he thought this might be one step toward repairing things with her. We did one session and he responded beautifully. No cravings. No withdrawal. That was it for the cigarettes. Just like that. He couldn't believe it.

Next he asked me if he could use hypnosis to get over the intimidation of cold-calling people. Again, we did this in one session. I helped him to see every call as an opportunity for success rather than failure. Now he loves cold-calling people. He does it for four hours every day and enjoys every minute of it because he has a new picture for it. He sees it in a new light.

Finally John told me that he was ready to deal with his struggle with food. Based on his response to the first two sessions we'd had, I thought changing his relationship to food—particularly stress-related eating—would be a snap. But we went through my standard two-session treatment process and nothing happened. John saw absolutely no change in his relationship with food. He was puzzled. I, on the other hand, was curious. Something in his mind was obviously preventing the pattern from breaking. What was scary about being lean, strong, and healthy? What did John think would happen? From other conversations, I knew that when he was in his late teens and early twenties he had been a lifeguard and incredibly fit. So I asked him, "What would happen if you looked like you did when you were twenty?"

It turns out that John was afraid that if he became thin, he would have an affair. He confessed that he and his wife had not slept in the same bed for more than a year, and he was afraid that if he lost weight, women would be attracted to him (even at 100 pounds overweight he was good-looking) and he would be vulnerable to their advances. He didn't want to do that to his wife or to his kids. I told him I understood, but that he was already having an affair with food and if he didn't do something about it soon, it was going to kill him, which would mean abandoning his wife and kids forever. I also pointed out that he was an adult and could make adult choices, meaning that if he was attracted to a woman or a woman made a pass at him, he was old enough and strong enough to know that an affair, like overeating, is a choice. Moreover, he had made the choice to stop smoking and he had. He had made the decision to change his mind about cold-calling and he had. After this conversation, John realized that the fantasy of his having an affair was just a way to rationalize his overeating. In reality, he loved his wife and did not want to cheat on her.

With this new understanding, we went through the same two-session treatment we had used the first time through. This time John responded beautifully. Within a year and a half, he lost the 100 pounds and got into incredible shape. He recently called to tell me that while he's not sure if the marriage is going to ultimately work out, he has been able to put real effort into the relationship and that his greatest reward is that he is able to be a better father. He bikes, runs, plays, and does schoolwork with his kids, strengthening and solidifying those bonds.

Many of my clients are like John and arrive at their first session with fears about what might happen if they actually lose weight. And like John, more often than not, their fears are their mind's trick to keep them in the never-ending fight with food.

The only time I encounter a fear of losing weight that is tied to a legitimate reality is when a client has been abused or sexually assaulted or has suffered from severe trauma. In these specific cases, the client has gained the weight as a kind of emotional protection. For instance, I have seen many men and women who have been raped or sexually abused gain weight after the experience to protect themselves from having it happen again. Their subconscious minds believe that the less attractive they are, the less likely they are to attract any kind of sexual advance. Sometimes this notion is clearly conscious as well, though it has no logical basis.

If you have been raped or physically or sexually abused or have suffered from severe trauma, then I strongly suggest that you see a psychiatrist or medical doctor before using medical hypnosis. These are deep, painful, and profound experiences that must be explored and understood before they can be released. It has been my experience that a client will not lose weight until he or she has dealt with all the issues surrounding these kinds of trauma.

The 4 percent of people who do not respond to clinical hypnosis typically have deeper underlying issues that food psychologically helps alleviate.* That said, if you find as you get deeper into this process that you do fall into this category and do not respond to the first or second scripts, then know that there is probably something that is keeping

---

*This statistic reflects my personal success rate within my practice. Therefore, statistics will vary by practice and practitioner.

you or has kept you from making a commitment to change. For most people, this deeper issue can be addressed with regular talk therapy, and then medical hypnosis can be effective.

Are You Ready?

Beyond our general fear of change, there are many obstacles—people, places, and things—that make it difficult for us to embrace change, even when it is for our own good.

Here are the thirteen most common things that prevent medical hypnosis from being as effective and as powerful as it can be:

1. You are doing this for someone else.

Who bought this book? If it was not you, did you borrow it? Or was it given to you? If it was given to you, how did you feel about receiving it? Did you feel insulted? Humiliated? Angry? When my mom dragged me to the doctor's office to talk to him about my weight and what we should do about it, all I wanted to do was eat more. Of course, I realize that my mom was only trying to help, but I was not ready to deal with my weight issue. When I was growing up, as much as I wanted to be thin and please my mother and attract girls, food was my salve, and I needed it to get through my teenage years. Only when food stopped working and I started feeling awful on a daily basis did I become open and ready to make the changes for me.

It's my experience that trying to lose weight for someone else never works. Not for your mother or your father or your siblings or your children. Not even for your partner. This is something that you need to do for you. Right here, right now, you need to decide whether or not you want to do this for you and whether you are really ready for what might be the biggest change of your life—no more food struggle, losing weight, feeling better, being free. This is huge. If you're feeling hesitant, maybe you are not committed 100 percent and you should put this book down until your own happiness rather than the happiness of others is your top priority. Think about it.

2. You are not or don't feel ready.

Of the thousands of clients who come to see me, I'd say roughly three in ten walk into my office and announce that they are not sure that they are ready for this. They are just there to talk and find out more about medical hypnosis. They tell me they want to do it after their closets are cleaned, after they move into a new house, when their kids are older, after they break up with so-and-so, once they've found their true love, after they get a raise or change jobs or stop working or start working or join a gym, when their life is more organized. All I can say about this is what I always say to them: Being ready for this kind of change is like being ready to have children. You never are totally ready. At some point you just have to look yourself in the mirror and say, "Yes," and dive into the process.

Furthermore, in my experience, when a person's out-of-control eating is addressed, then everything in that person's life gets better. When you are healthier, you have more energy, time, and ability to focus on the other areas of your life. The house gets organized. The promotion becomes a reality. The relationship deepens. I know this from my own personal experience and from watching thousands of clients' lives get better once they've addressed their unhealthy minds.

3. You don't think you are worth it.

How many times have you told yourself with your inner voice or said out loud, "I'm worthless," "I'm a failure," or some variation of these statements?

My client Anita is an excellent example of someone who never valued her life and watched her health deteriorate because of it. When forty-five-year-old Anita came to see me she had four kids and a husband who worked eighty to a hundred hours a week. Anita was only 10 pounds overweight, but she was suffering from high blood pressure, high cholesterol, and high stress, which she felt was going to lead to cancer—a disease nearly everyone in her family has or had—any day.

I asked her what was going on. She told me she had no time to eat healthfully. Making sure that the family was taken care of was more important. She was constantly running around, carpooling the kids, feeding the kids, making sure her husband was happy, and keeping the house clean and the laundry under control. She confessed that all she ate was junk food: corn chips, pretzels, the kids' leftover lunch snacks, and soda—the typical mother-of-young-children diet drill.

I told Anita that she needed to start putting herself first. She told me she didn't want to be selfish and that for her the kids came first. I told her that being a healthy mother was not selfish—rather, being healthy and happy was an excellent model for her children and that she would be of no help to her family if she got sick. She said, "Well, if you put it like that, I see your point. But I still have no time!"

We talked about what would be a feasible solution given her time constraints. First, we came up with several easy strategies for her to get lean protein and vegetables into her diet without spending hours in the kitchen. From there on out, along with buying groceries for her kids and husband, Anita would stock her kitchen with turkey slices, bits of grilled chicken, tofu, cut-up carrots and broccoli, fruit, and other healthy foods that were easy to grab on the go. We also talked about doing a few five-minute mini meditations throughout the day (I will show you how to do this in Chapter 12). This would help Anita relax and be less inclined to eat poorly if she were running late or if the kids were acting out. As soon as Anita started doing these mini meditations and changing the food in her cupboards and refrigerator, she lost the 10 pounds, had more energy, and felt better. Anita had not been in a struggle with food as much as in a struggle with herself. She needed to learn that taking care of herself was not a selfish act, that putting herself first was actually a way of taking care of her family, and that she was worth it.

Likewise, this process is about you valuing yourself and your life. You need to put yourself first. You need to believe you are worth it. Binging and overeating do not make you a bad person. They make you a person who has a conflict between the conscious mind, which wants to be healthy and lean, and the subconscious mind, which has been programmed to overeat. You are good, no matter what. And you are worth it, no matter how old, sick, or overweight you are. If you believe in this process and yourself, you can change.

4. You think it is too late.

It is never too late. I have had clients in their seventies and eighties come to see me to address their struggle with food and to reverse conditions such as heart disease and type II diabetes. Medical hypnosis can also help manage blood pressure and ease the pain of arthritis, which is aggravated by excessive weight.

A few years ago, a special-education teacher named Kathy walked into my office. She was sixty-four years old, was more than 100 pounds overweight, and had extremely high blood pressure and type II diabetes. She actually had a fairly healthy diet except for her obsession with gumdrops. She ate roughly eight or nine large bags of them a week and carried them with her everywhere—in the car, in her briefcase, in her pockets. Kathy was adding an extra 6,500 calories a week, including 1,931 grams of sugar, to her diet just with those gumdrops! This exacerbated her diabetes, and she was experiencing severe joint pain and backaches.

I asked her if this gumdrop habit had been a lifelong obsession or if it was new. She told me that she had started eating them when her husband died, roughly a year and a half before. I asked her if it had been a painful loss. She told me that it had actually been a relief: Her husband had physically abused her and she had always been too scared to leave the marriage. After telling her how sorry I was to know this, I pointed out that she had managed to continue the abuse. "How so?" she asked, and I replied, "By eating so much sugar that you are in physical pain."

Her eyes widened and she burst into tears. "Oh my God, you're right! I can't believe I'm doing to myself exactly what he did to me."

After she'd recognized the roots of her behavior, we used medical hypnosis to create a new, self-loving tape in her head. We created a script that told her that she would care for herself as she would for any precious life. When I saw Kathy six months later, she confessed that she had also been cutting herself for nearly forty years but had finally stopped. The new self-love wiring had not only healed the overeating but also stopped a lifelong hurtful habit. Moreover, Kathy lost more than 100 pounds in fourteen months and now swims three or four days a week. After she lost the weight, she called to tell me, "I didn't think

I could have a new life at sixty-five, but I do and it is truly amazing."

With the Alpha Solution, you can change your mind at any time. Nonetheless, you should keep in mind that the longer the thinking and behavior have been in place, the longer it typically takes to change them. You will notice changes in the first two weeks, but it may take time to permanently change the habit. As you saw with Kathy, it took her six months to change a forty-year habit of cutting, whereas her gumdrop obsession, which was relatively short-lived, took less time.

5. You don't believe it can work for you.

If you're reading all this and thinking, "This can't be true. I can't get better after all these years. Dr. Glassman doesn't know me or my story. I'm different," you're probably wrong. Unless you have suffered a severe trauma that has inspired an unhealthy relationship with food, you can change your food blueprint using the methods in this book.

This said, the more you have told yourself you cannot do something or that you are not worth it over the years, the stronger that pattern has become in your brain. Undoing it may be harder, but it is not impossible. If, like my client Kathy, you start saying positive things to yourself and establishing and building a new self-loving pattern for living, someday that pattern will override the old pattern and you will win. As you will learn in Chapter 4, we become what our inner voice tells us. For instance, I recently heard a celebrity who was very vocal about her gastric bypass surgery say, after gaining back 55 pounds, "I just know I am always going to be plagued with this struggle with food." If your inner voice is a broken record of self-loathing statements, it is easy to recognize the real monster in your struggle. Likewise, if you think positive, loving thoughts about yourself, your inner voice will be your ally and anything is possible.

6. You are ambivalent about or scared of using medical hypnosis.

Unfortunately, because the success of medical hypnosis rests very much on the patterns of the mind, it can be hampered if you are determinedly skeptical and don't believe it can help you.

I once had a client who was referred to me by his doctor but was terrified because his priest had told him that if he used hypnosis, the devil would enter him. While this might sound silly to many of us, he was truly scared. As with all my clients, I explained to him that a hypnotic state is natural and that we experience it several times a day every day, and that a hypnotic state is the same thing as a meditative state. But he could not get past the idea of some horrible force entering his body. So, in the end, he could not and did not use medical hypnosis, and to my knowledge, he never ended his struggle with food, which in my opinion was the real devil.

But I've also had many clients who have come in to see me and are initially scared, yet they go on to overcome their fear and have great success. For instance, my client Charlotte called me a few years ago. I had worked with her and her husband a few years prior and they'd had great success; now they wanted me to work with their housekeeper, Gloria. I asked why she was calling instead of Gloria. She explained that five years ago, Gloria had choked on a piece of tuna fish and almost died. Her husband had saved her life by performing the Heimlich maneuver, but since then she had become increasingly scared of eating for fear of choking on food. First she wouldn't eat tuna. Then it became anything that had the texture of the tuna salad she had been eating at the time—egg salad, chicken salad. Then it became not eating any animal products. Then it became a fear of bread. Five years later, she was hospitalized and dying because she was not eating. Charlotte had encouraged Gloria's husband to get help. They had consulted doctors, psychiatrists, and therapists to no avail. Then Charlotte realized that medical hypnosis, which had helped her stop overeating, might be able to help Gloria start eating. So she called me. And I said, "It probably can. Let's give it a shot."

When I went to see Gloria in the hospital, she was as scared as my client with the priest had been. As a devout Catholic from Ecuador, she also thought manipulating the mind was the devil's playground. But she trusted her employers, Charlotte and Bill, and saw that they had been changed only for the positive by medical hypnosis (both had lost more than 50 pounds each). And after talking to me she realized that she wanted to live more than she wanted to die, so she decided to give medical hypnosis a go.

We reframed her traumatic experience so that her brain's wiring conceived of the event as something that happened long ago and associated the act of eating with something silly. So instead of associating eating with choking, she now saw eating as a funny and fun experience.

To the shock of her husband and the doctors, the very day we did the reframing and associating, Gloria started eating again. Three weeks later, she'd gained 10 pounds. After several months in the hospital, she was allowed to go home. Today, she is healthy, back at work, and eating everything and anything except tuna fish, which is only natural given her experience with it.

All of this is to say that if you're really scared, then maybe medical hypnosis is not for you. But my guess is that, like most of my clients, once you experience the deep relaxation and power of the alpha state, there will be no going back.

7. Someone around you likes you, maybe even needs you, to be fat.

I cannot tell you how many clients I've seen whose partner, mother, father, sister, brother, or even friend likes the fact that the person carries a few extra pounds. Some jealous men and women secretly or subconsciously prefer their partner to carry a few extra pounds because they think the partner is then less likely to attract others or have affairs. So they sabotage the partner's attempt to be lean, strong, and healthy. Mothers, sisters, and friends become competitive and don't want their daughter, sister, or friend looking better than they do. Fathers don't want men coming near their daughters. Brothers don't want their brothers getting the girls they can't get. This sabotage comes in many forms.

After you've announced that you are going to lose some weight, has your partner, spouse, mother, father, or friend ever made it difficult for you to go to the gym, encouraged you to overeat, or brought home donuts, chocolates, your favorite cheese, or a cake? If so, then you've got someone who, on some level, is scared of you realizing your true physical, emotional, and mental potential. Before you go any further, you must sit this person down and explain that you are doing this for yourself and that he or she must respect this. If the person doesn't, then he or she is not loving you in a truly loving way. Supporting some-one's unhealthy habits is not caring or kind.

If you cannot have this conversation, or if your partner, parent, sib-ling, or friend has an adverse reaction to this conversation, then you must know that you are not likely to succeed in losing weight and becoming lean, strong, and healthy because there will be a conflict. You will feel like you can either get the love from the person who is close to you or lose weight and lose that person. This is a painful, sometimes excruciating choice to make. In my experience, more often than not, we will seek love, even if it is unhealthy love, over our own health and well-being. All I can say about this is that there are other kinds of love out there. If you recognize this as your situation, I strongly recommend that you see a therapist who specializes in weight and self-esteem issues. This is a complicated relationship to unravel.

8. You are a self-saboteur.

Are you the kind of person who gets only so far in a job or on a project and then does something to keep yourself from being promoted or fin-ishing the project? Do you always seem to have a glass ceiling over you? Are you ambivalent about what you want? I am a firm believer that there are no accidents. We don't just forget meetings, to call, or to do things. We don't do them for a reason.

I want you to think about the ways in which you may have sabotaged yourself and your weight-loss success over the years. Did you decide to go on a diet and then agree to meet friends at your favorite place for binging the next day? Do you buy unhealthy foods when you know you should not? Do you keep putting down this book or leaving it at home when you planned on reading it on your lunch hour?

If you have been sabotaging your success, you've got to figure out why you feel you don't deserve happiness. What is your glass ceiling? What is keeping you from breaking through? Why are you allowing yourself to get so far and then trip up? How is not succeeding working for you?

9. You are addicted to suffering.

It might sound crazy to suggest this—after all, who enjoys suffering?—but being addicted to feeling pain is a common roadblock for many of my clients. For some people, pain is a way to feel alive. It is the only sensation they can feel.

As I mentioned earlier, part of my journey to being ready to commit to losing weight was letting go of the idea that my life was about a painful fight with food. You might be thinking, "No way. That's not me. I want to be happy." But I'd like you to think hard about this idea of needing suffering in your life. There are many different kinds of suffering. For instance, I had a lonely client who kept eating because it made her sick and then she had to go to the doctor's office, where she would be around people. I've had countless clients who liked the attention that being overweight got them, even if it was negative attention. Give yourself a moment to think about this. Is there any reason why being in a fight with food works for you? Does it keep people away? Does it keep your partner away and you like this because you do not enjoy sex (or at least having sex with him or her)? Does it distract you from other life issues you do not want to address? Does it draw attention to you? Remember: Negative attention ("You shouldn't eat so much") is still attention. Do you secretly like the attention that doctors give you? Do you do it to keep someone angry or disappointed in you? Do you do it because your mother, father, or sibling overeats or binges and you feel it is the only way to bond to or connect with that person (think: hanging out on the couch eating pizza)? Do you eat and eat because you have given up on the idea that you can be as attractive or as successful as your thin sister or brother? Do you stay overweight to punish someone else?

These may seem like odd and intrusive questions, but you need to answer them honestly. If these questions are not explored (best done with a well-qualified and experienced therapist), then you may be limiting your ability to use medical hypnosis to its maximum strength and healing capacity.

10. Playing the blame game.

Whose fault is it that you are engaged in a struggle with food? Mom? Dad? Your brother? Sister? Aunt? Uncle? Grandparent? Friend? Foe? More than likely, the answer is all of the above.

So maybe you were overfed as a child. Or maybe your father never let you eat candy, so it became an obsession as an adult. Maybe you snacked on your mother's homemade cookies when studying for exams during high school and now any cookie is your preferred antidote to all kinds of stress. Of course it is of immense value to understand where our patterns emerge from, and in Chapter 5 we will explore the classic parent/child and sibling/sibling patterns and how they evolve. But no matter what the roots of the problem are, you need to realize that

YOU ARE ULTIMATELY RESPONSIBLE.

Who is putting the food in your mouth?

YOU.

Even though when you overeat, snack, or binge you may feel possessed by a large, powerful force and feel like you have no other choice but to eat, you need to know that it is you who is reaching for that food and swallowing it. So from here on out, you have a choice. Either you can blame the world and your mother for your woes, or you can take your life back into your own hands and get well. The first step: Make the choice to not blame someone else for your problem. You should never let anyone else's voice have more power than your own.

11. You suffer from the f*ck-its.

In my experience, people who suffer from what I call the "f*ck-its" are related to the people who like to blame; they just do the blaming in broader strokes. Instead of blaming their father for their problems, they blame the world.

My client Peter is a classic example of someone who suffered from the f*ck-its. He came to me on the first anniversary of the September 11 terrorist attacks. He worked for Cantor Fitzgerald, one of the New York City firms that was hardest hit by the attack on the World Trade Center. His firm lost 658 people in one day, which was absolutely devastating. Peter was on vacation at the time, and his guilt for not being there and for surviving was overwhelming.

Until September 11 happened, Peter had struggled with the same 25 pounds for about fifteen years. He went to the gym and tried to eat well, but stress snacking kept the 25 pounds on. After September 11, however, he asked himself, "Why am I bothering to try to lose weight when the world is such a mess? Why should I even try?" In a year, Peter went from being 25 pounds overweight to being 100 pounds overweight.

When Peter came to see me, I recognized his situation as a classic case of post-traumatic stress. Until September 11, 2001, Peter had viewed the world as a good place. He felt proud to have brought three children into the world. But after September 11, all Peter saw when he looked around him was suffering (the loss of 658 people) and terror (the fear that it could happen to him and his children). He told me that he felt the floor had fallen out from under him. I agreed that it had. But I also pointed out to him that he was still alive and his f*ck-it attitude was not only affecting him but was also hurting his children and family.

Because Peter's overeating had more to do with the trauma of September 11, I told him that I didn't think he needed medical hypnosis. He needed something to help him deal with his upset and stress. I taught him how to meditate, which is hypnosis without the use of suggestion. Meditation is the best exercise I know for reducing stress and bolstering positive thinking. In his daily meditation, there was nothing about food; instead it focused on relaxation and practicing self-love for mind and body. It was a way for Peter to get his head ready for the day, to focus and to start out optimistically, to think about and visualize every positive aspect of his life.

Within three months, Peter was back at the gym and feeling alive for the first time since that horrible September day. In a year, he lost all the weight, including the 25 pounds he had been struggling with for fifteen years. People in his office were so blown away by this transformation that twenty others from the firm came to see me.

Like Peter, most people who suffer from the f*ck-its have good reason for feeling this way. Perhaps someone died or left suddenly. Or maybe, out of the blue, something really awful happened to you or a family member. Maybe you simply live or work in a place where there is suffering. There's a reason why I see so many nurses, doctors, and lawyers. When you spend twelve to sixteen hours a day in a stressful environment watching people in pain and dying or helping them negotiate the pain in their life, it changes your attitude.

Nonetheless, having the f*ck-its ultimately hurts only you and those close to you. And there are better ways of dealing with the darker sides of our modern reality. Like meditating. Like volunteering somewhere. Like spending time with the ones we love doing constructive activities, from knitting to biking to going to a concert. Sometimes after a long day, my wife and I go for a drive or walk around our neighborhood, which is adjacent to a county reserve, and that is enough to bring me back, to make me remember the joy of living. Even a five-minute mini meditation can offer release.

12. You are incapable of being honest with yourself.

Part of the medical hypnosis process is taking an inventory. If you are not honest about what you are eating, how much you are eating, and how you are eating, then the hypnosis session you create for yourself will not help you all that much. How honest are you being with yourself in your Life Log? This is as good a gauge as anything. You will succeed only as much as you let yourself succeed. If you are rigorously honest, you will get substantial results.

13. You are confusing awareness with action.

Okay, so you have admitted you are in a struggle with food. This is a good first step. But awareness is not enough. As you well know, saying "I am an overeater" or "I am a binger" does not cause you to immediately start shedding pounds. Nor does beating yourself up for being in a struggle with food. Even in the world of machines, it's not the mechanics that get the results, it's the action. Similarly, the actions you will undertake with the help of this book will make your brain operate properly. Through using medical hypnosis, you will teach your brain to have a healthy eating mind, which will in turn help you lose weight and become lean, strong, and healthy.

No matter how much you weigh—if you want to lose and keep off 5 or 50 or 150 pounds—you can do it. I'll be honest, it takes work. But if after reading all of this you feel ready, then let's begin.

The Alpha Solution

Chapter Three

> To change one's mind is rather a sign of
> prudence than ignorance.
>
> —Spanish proverb

Crystals, feathers, pocket watches, metronomes, rituals, the occult, trance-inducing words or phrases, feeling groggy or like you are in an altered state, being out of control, walking around like a zombie—these things have *nothing* to do with hypnosis. They have to do with misrepresentations of hypnosis in popular culture. The hypnosis you see in films like *The Curse of the Jade Scorpion* or *The Manchurian Candidate* is not hypnosis. It's material invented to entertain you, as is the hypnosis you see on magicians' stages and in nightclub acts.

Yet hypnotic or trance states themselves are not Hollywood creations. Trance or hypnosis is a scientifically proven natural state of consciousness that *everyone* experiences *every day*. Believe it or not, you have already experienced hypnosis thousands of times in your life.

What Is Medical Hypnosis?

All human brains produce electrical activity, and the level of electrical activity determines our state of consciousness—from wide awake to deep sleep. Our general, awake, fully operating state is called the beta state; this is when the brain is producing electrical activity at about 20 cycles per second. You are in beta as you are reading this (unless you are zoning out, in which case you are not!). You are in beta when you talk. Essentially, you are in beta when you are interacting with the world, from grocery shopping to writing a letter.

When the brain slows down a little and produces approximately 8–14 cycles of electrical activity per second, a person is in the alpha-dominant state. I consider this to be our body's natural trance or hypnotic state. Examples of this alpha state are daydreaming, boredom, when you are just waking up, practicing yoga or any exercise like tai chi where breathing is emphasized, zoning out while driving on the highway, feeling mesmerized by a movie or a book, falling asleep, or meditating. (Contrary to popular understanding, meditation is not a religion. It is actually the same state as hypnosis. Meditation is just hypnosis without the use of suggestion.) Our everyday hypnotic or trance states are the times during the day when we feel relaxed and lost in an experience or thought.

All humans also experience a hypnotic or trance state every night, beginning when they are lying in bed, zoning out, and feeling relaxed and ready to make the transition from awake to asleep. When this happens you're actually in a trance, a very deep hypnotic state.

Other levels of brain activity include the deeper levels of sleep: theta, delta, and rapid eye movement (REM). When in theta, which follows the alpha state, the brain is slower, cycling 6–8 times per second. The early theta state is a deep hypnotic state. Delta is when our brains are cycling 4–5 times per second and is a very deep level of sleep. As you can see, the deeper the level of sleep you are in, the slower your brain activity is. The delta state is also a transitional state that happens when our brains are on their way to REM sleep, where they cycle only 3 or 4 times per second.

Because the alpha state is the bridge between our conscious state (being awake) and our unconscious state (being asleep), many scientists have correlated the alpha state to when the subconscious mind is especially receptive to words and images. I agree. Hundreds of thousands of cases where people have used hypnosis and suggestion to heal, alleviate pain, and change their minds during the last two hundred years show us not only that this is true, but also that the alpha state is the best state for accessing, watching, and talking to the subconscious mind.

When I use the term *subconscious mind,* I'm not talking about the Freudian definition that describes our subconscious minds as warehouses for our repressed and painful memories. While many scientists suspect that Freud was right—that the subconscious mind is in fact a house for our memories—they also know that Freud's definition is limited. I use the term *subconscious mind* to represent that part of us that houses the blueprint for all of our behaviors, habits, tastes, and preferences.

Through using MRI and single photon emission computed tomography (SPECT) scans, scientists can track the brain's activity. In fact, measuring cognition has become so precise by means of the MRI that scientists can tell the difference between a brain that reacts to one kind of product packaging versus another. Imagine the impact this will have on market research!

But what's even more spectacular is the fact that scientists have not only discovered the patterns and behaviors associated with stimuli such as colors and smells but have also determined that every human's brain has a particular electrical pattern or blueprint for every repeated interaction the person has with his or her environment. This means that an electrical pattern is established for how we experience books, food, exercise, feet, fashion—you name it and your brain has a blueprint for it. These behaviors and habits are established during a person's early development and, through repetition, reflect and direct that person's habits and behaviors for the rest of his or her life.

Think about someone you find offensive. Picture yourself riding in a hot car with him or her for three hours. Feel the disgust and rage rising within you? This feeling is stored in your subconscious mind. Likewise, think about a food that you love. Picture yourself pulling that food out of the pantry or refrigerator. Imagine putting it on a plate. See yourself eating it. You might already be salivating. This is the power of your imagination and your subconscious mind's blueprint. A mere thought produces a patterned physiological response.

The subconscious mind's reactions I've just described are the natural and normal reactions of a healthy brain. But the subconscious mind can also be trained to have unhealthy inclinations. For instance, if a person's brain has a blueprint for binging on Oreo cookies when upset, the binging will become a repeat occurrence because the subconscious mind has been patterned for this. This kind of blueprint is what leads to unhealthy cravings, snacking, overeating, and ultimately weight gain.

It is no accident that scientists named this level of electrical brain activity with the first letter of the Greek alphabet. *Alpha* means the beginning. Our subconscious mind is our beginning—the beginning of what defines us as unique, individual human beings. If your subconscious mind was trained at an early age to be an overeating mind, this is where the pattern was established and will remain. The only way to stop overeating is to change your mind. Literally.

When we are in the alpha state, our subconscious mind—the place where our food preferences and behaviors are stored—is most receptive to suggestion, new ideas, and change. This is why it is important for people to pay attention to what they're doing and who and what's around them during the time just before and as they fall asleep. In these few minutes, any outside stimuli have particular access to our subconscious mind, from a conversation to music to what's on the television. Have you ever fallen asleep watching someone eat a hot dog on television and woken up the next day with an unbelievable hankering for a hot dog? This is because the television had direct access to your subconscious mind. Falling asleep to a horror flick on TV will also influence your dreams, even disrupt your sleep. And this is why the old marriage adage to never go to bed angry is something worth listening to.

When we use medical hypnosis for behavior modification and habit adjustment, we rely on this same receptivity, but harness the power of our suggestibility and neuroplasticity for the good health and well-being of a person—reframing unhealthy habits to become healthy ones. **At its heart, hypnosis is a creative visualization process supported by language.**

As we've discussed, early in life your mind acquires a food blueprint. Medical hypnosis helps the brain reimagine or renovate the parts of your "house" that don't function properly, providing your brain with a new picture to follow. It's like asking your brain to reenvision the image of a cube sitting on one of its flat sides on a table to see the cube spinning on one of its corners. This transition process is called reframing. It's still a cube, but it's a cube that's been tweaked to appear differently.

The power of the brain's imagination is not to be underestimated. Remember your mouth salivating just because you thought of a favorite food? That is your imagination at work. And when scientists put this notion of imagination producing cravings and physiological reactions to the test, it was established as a proven fact. For example, when an alcoholic is shown a picture of a cocktail on a video screen while his brain is being scanned, technicians can actually see the craving response begin. But even more remarkable is that the same craving response kicks in when the alcoholic is asked to simply think about a cocktail. What's even more astonishing about this is that when scientists repeated the same test—showing a picture and then just asking the person to use their imagination—with other behaviors they found that the *exact* same craving reaction appeared on their MRI pictures. Scientists did more studies and found that the only other thing to cause this powerful craving reaction was a person's sense of smell, which is our most powerful sense. This means that our imagination is as strong as our most powerful and primal sense. More than our intuition, our imagination is truly our sixth sense. So if we can use our imagination to provoke our most primal physical and emotional responses, then we can certainly use our imagination to reframe a physiological response to certain foods.

For instance, perhaps you have a three o'clock snacking problem where every day you crave a sugary or salty snack at three (assuming you're not diabetic or hypoglycemic). This might be due to the fact that when you were young your mother provided you with an after-school snack as soon as you came in the door, which was around three o'clock. When it comes to general programming, such as with eating, the brain is very straightforward: Like any and every other muscle and organ in our bodies, its cells get trained to work one way. If you were to then use medical hypnosis, you would slow the mind down to an alpha state and talk to the subconscious mind to create a new association with three o'clock. Maybe you'd picture a full stomach or an apple instead of 1,680 calories' worth of Doritos and a 300-calorie soda, or a 160-calorie skim latte instead of a 550-calorie medium Strawberry Banana Smoothie from Dunkin' Donuts.[1,2]

Beyond swapping foods for other foods, medical hypnosis also uses the imagination to make the problem smaller using visualization. The first of the three steps of the Alpha Solution is a Release, which essentially tells the subconscious mind to let old patterns and habits go. The Release uses the imagination to tell the brain to picture shrinking and destroying a box containing all the old messages. This visualization actually convinces the subconscious mind that the box and everything in it—food, behaviors, problems—are gone. As we will discuss in Chapter 4, the subconscious accepts this because it does not know the difference between fantasy and reality. Essentially, the subconscious mind will go for this imagined reality hook, line, and sinker because it "saw" it happen. As a result, whatever was put into that box is removed. The unhealthy blueprint is addressed and put in its proper place.

Likewise, the second and third steps of the Alpha Solution, Reframing and Reinforcing, also use the imagination to introduce new, healthy eating habits and behaviors to the subconscious mind. When you repeatedly present an imagined picture of yourself eating properly to your subconscious mind while you are in the alpha state, a new, healthy food blueprint is formed. We will talk more about the Reframing and Reinforcing steps later in the chapter, but before we move on, let's get back to the facts about medical hypnosis.

When you are in a hypnotic alpha state, you are not asleep. You are more awake, more focused, more absorbed, and more relaxed than usual.

Just because you are not in beta, our brain's fastest-cycling state, does not mean you are somewhere else. Think about how you feel when you daydream or are hypnotically driving along a highway. The world seems irrelevant, right? This is because you are internally focused, exploring ideas, fantasies, and feelings, rather than externally focused on the people or things around you. This does not mean that you are not alert or awake. It means that you are absorbed in and by your mind. This internal focus is actually a heightened state of consciousness because you are watching your mind—its thoughts, thought patterns, and habits.

This ability to focus on our thoughts, feelings, and habits is a natural and powerful tool that techniques such as medical hypnosis and meditation optimize. For instance, I have a client who meditates regularly. When she first started, she observed that whenever she had an uncomfortable thought while meditating—fear of getting older, worries about her son, recalling a fight with her husband—she thought about food next: guilt about what she'd eaten before she sat down to meditate, what she was going to eat after she meditated, fantasies about eating only bread and chocolate cake for the rest of her life and never getting fat. She soon realized that her brain thought of food as a salve for her fears. This awareness led her to become aware of her brain's trigger response to reach for a carbohydrate whenever she was nervous or upset. Her ability to use the alpha state to look internally at her subconscious mind helped her to stop a lifelong struggle.

You are in control at all times.

Fact: No one can control you unless you let them. Therefore, no one can control another person using hypnosis. The idea that when you are in a hypnotic state, you are susceptible to others' wills and whims stems from the very false notion that hypnosis is something that is done *to* someone, rather than a healthy, naturally occurring state.

All hypnosis is self-hypnosis.

Because the hypnotic or alpha state is a natural state, only you can ask your brain's electrical activity to slow down to alpha. All I do as a therapist is facilitate the process. This means that I provide my clients with instructions that hundreds of years of practice have shown to be effective in helping a person slow the brain's electrical activity down. These instructions are not complicated—I simply ask my clients to picture themselves feeling relaxed, comfortable, and at ease. There are no magic words or methods; it's a simple process. This is why it is possible for me to put my techniques in a book and for you to be able to use it safely and effectively on your own.

However, it is important that people be willing and open to the idea of slowing their brain down or they will not effectively enter the alpha state for the purpose of behavior modification. People who might have a hard time slowing their brains down are those who suffer from obsessive-compulsive disorder, attention deficit disorder, or a physical tic. These challenges make it harder for the person to concentrate and physically relax.

During hypnosis you don't lose your sense of right and wrong.

As much as your subconscious mind rules your behaviors and actions, your conscious mind rules your world of right and wrong. So your subconscious mind will do only what your conscious mind will allow. This means that if any suggestion to your subconscious mind conflicts with your conscious beliefs—from a belief in God to a belief that murder is wrong—you will reject the conflicting suggestion. For instance, if you were in a trance state and someone—a therapist, friend, or foe—were to suggest that you leave the office, rob a bank, and bring the money back, you would reject this suggestion because, unless you are a professional bank robber, you consciously know that robbing a bank is wrong. In fact, a disturbing suggestion such as this would probably invite more brain activity, moving your brain from its alpha state to the high-functioning beta state, and you would tell the therapist, friend, or foe that he or she was crazy, then leave. So don't worry—essentially, if a suggestion isn't kosher, you're not going to accept it.

Medical hypnosis is not new.

Medical hypnosis, also known as clinical hypnosis or hypnotherapy, is a therapeutic application approved by the American Psychological Association and the American Medical Association and utilized by cognitive/behavioral therapists and other health providers. The American Medical Association approved of medical hypnosis in 1958, so this is not a new practice by any means. It has been studied and practiced for centuries by tens of thousands of physicians, psychologists, mental health professionals, dentists, registered nurses, dermatologists, and laypeople. Harvard University scientists were among the first to use rigorous clinical studies to analyze what happens in the meditative states of monks. Decades later, in August 2003, *Time* magazine published an MRI of the brain in the meditative state.[3]

Medical hypnosis is safe.

Unlike other diet approaches where the body is stressed, starved, and sublimated, there are no side effects or dangers with hypnosis. Remember, it occurs naturally and it is safe, effective, and relatively easy. The medicinal benefits of clinical hypnosis have been documented in hundreds of academic studies and some of the world's top universities and medical centers. It is practiced by health care providers associated with or on staff at such illustrious institutions as Memorial Sloan-Kettering, Columbia, Brown, Yale, Harvard, Rutgers, Mt. Sinai, Duke, Stanford, and hundreds of others in the United States alone. Hypnosis clinicians are also affiliated with thousands of hospital burn centers and cancer treatment programs throughout the world.

Medical hypnosis is widely applied.

Beyond treating overeating, hypnosis has also been a proven and invaluable technique for the treatment of smoking cessation, eating disorders, anxiety, concentration, insomnia, phobias, pain control, stuttering, post-traumatic stress disorder, and performance enhancement. In fact, I work with many world-class athletes, including key members of the most successful major league teams, some of the world's top-ranked tennis players, leading concert musicians, and famous stage and screen actors, as well as top amateur gymnasts, and even weekend tennis buffs and golfers.

Your ability to experience hypnosis has nothing to do with intelligence, race, age, gender, or willpower.

As I've said, *everyone* experiences the alpha state. Therefore *everyone* can harness this natural human ability for healing. Drs. Herbert Spiegel and David Spiegel, men who have done extensive research on medical hypnosis and are leaders in the field, say there "is no difference in hypnotizability of women compared to men."[4] Likewise, there is no distinction made according to race, class, or age. This said, as a therapist, I have a responsibility to protect and warn two groups of people who should not use medical hypnosis without the supervision of a therapist: those who have been diagnosed with a serious mental illness and those who have endured the trauma of rape and/or sexual abuse. In these particular cases, special considerations will be necessary.

For nearly everyone who is overweight, overeats, has cravings, nocturnally binges, or is thin but struggles with the pull of certain foods such as chocolate or bread, medical hypnosis is the permanent answer to their food fight.

If every cell in your body wants to be thin but you still have overpowering cravings, eat large portions, or snack on unhealthy foods such as McDonald's, Coke, pizza, or chocolate, then you have an out-of-shape, fat brain and no diet or diet food is going to work. Why? Because diet programs deal only with the food you're eating, not the person eating the food and the underlying neuropathways for these foods. They don't address the hardwired psychological desire to overeat, crave "feel-good" foods, or snack when there's no real need for food. As I said in Chapter 1, hundreds of studies by venerable institutions have shown that 95 percent of people who use weight-loss programs cannot keep the weight off for more than a year. And more often than not, the 95 percent who regain the weight put back on more than they lost. These numbers are in stark contrast to the 96 percent of my clients who use my Lite-State Method practice of clinical hypnosis to change their relationship with food and lose the weight they want to lose—permanently and without a struggle. As you are learning, medical hypnosis is the only method that helps your subconscious mind to reframe the hardwiring so that you will want to make healthy food decisions to support and promote your body's well-being.

The Lite-State Method

All of us have a dream picture of ourselves and how we'd like to be in the world. When I was twenty, it was to be thinner and to have a career I would love and be good at. I now live my dream. So when I work with people, I believe it is my job to help them realize their dream—from making french fries have less appeal to losing 20 or 200 pounds.

I have studied, worked with, and practiced medical hypnosis for more than 25 years, honing my systems and tweaking the language, and have used my research and experience to develop my Lite-State Method of medical hypnosis. Several things distinguish my method from other approaches.

I treat one person at a time.

Many hypnosis practitioners use hypnosis in group settings where the group has a common goal: to stop smoking, say, or to lose weight. The problem with working this way is that the language they use is generic. For instance, imagine a mother who is carrying fifteen extra pounds and has a serious snacking problem due to a deep relationship with cashews. Now imagine her surrounded by fifty other men and women who want to lose weight, from 10 to 100 pounds. The practitioner's challenge is to find a way to meet all these people's needs. So, while talking to them, the practitioner must use general language. And when she gets to an issue such as snacking, she can only use a phrase as generic as "snack foods" to ensure that she's hitting everyone's issues. But, as you've learned, the subconscious mind is a very literal organ. If this woman's subconscious mind has no established association or relationship with the phrase "snack foods," these words will be meaningless and move on to other thoughts. This woman needs cashew language for her cashew problem.

The other problem with using medical hypnosis in groups is that the practitioner's generically scripted words will not be specific enough about the behaviors around the particular problem foods. Let's look again at our cashew example. If the mother craves cashews in her car on the way to pick up her children from school, then the practitioner's discussion and images of hanging on to a refrigerator door or passing the pantry are not going to help this woman's subconscious mind change because her snacking problem has no relationship or association to those behaviors. Her brain is going to say, "I eat cashews in the car and don't refrigerate my nuts. Speaking of nuts, you are driving me nuts! I'm outta here."

If this woman came to me and said, "I need to lose 15 pounds, which I gained when I was pregnant and keep on with a hard-core afternoon snack of a pound of cashews," I would work with her one-on-one to identify how to root out the specific behaviors and language that her subconscious mind would recognize and respond to. Likewise, in this book we will spend four chapters identifying the language and behaviors specific to your needs and habits so that your subconscious mind will respond and be receptive to change.

I treat one problem at a time.

While medical hypnosis can treat a wide range of issues, from purging to panic disorder, I address only one issue at a time. Why? Well, would you want a surgeon to perform heart and brain surgery on you at the same time? No, because it would be too traumatic and might kill you. While working on several issues at a time using medical hypnosis would not kill you, it would not serve you well or crack the patterns you're trying to break. As we've explored, these patterns are electrical relationships, and they are trained into your brain the same way your computer is trained to look for your home's wireless connection first. When we have a thought of a certain food, it triggers our brain's neurons to fire in a certain pattern. Medical hypnosis helps alter these patterns and sets new ones. But the brain can manage only so much interruption at a time or it overloads. When we address one problem at a time, it ensures that the changes we're making are effectively loaded, accepted, and used. There is no thought confusion. This is why this book addresses only food issues.

I am thorough. My Lite-State Method includes using the three steps—Release, Reframing, and Reinforcement—that have become the gold standard in the field.

Typically, I see clients for weight issues for two or three sessions, and I use different approaches for the first and second sessions. Why? Because the first session identifies the underlying food patterns and foods, determines a way to contain and release these issues, and focuses the person's subconscious mind on the idea of being rid of this struggle. Remember the shrinking box image? This is a first-session technique because we are making a food right-sized and smashing an old, unhealthy behavior to bits. In the second session, we use a different set of metaphors and pictures to reframe the client's relationship with food. The focus is on the fact that the client's food struggle has been contained (it's in a sealed box) and is now behind the client. And the client's Reinforcement of the Releasing and Reframing happens when he or she listens to a personalized CD, which strengthens the new, healthy picture of food: that food is fuel and that the client now eats in a way that promotes health and well-being.

My first appointment lasts for an hour. During this session I explain the medical hypnosis process in detail, educating my clients (as I will do with you in Chapter 4) about neuroplasticity and what medical hypnosis really is. Then I get a client's background information and learn his or her food story (as I will do with you in Chapter 5). I will ask the client when the struggle with food began, how the relationship has developed (usually, overeating starts as a general habit and the patterns get more specific and sophisticated as the person grows), and whether an eating behavior—binging, snacking, a powerful craving—has ever scared him or her. I will also ask the client why he or she has come to see me. What does the client want to do? Arrest powerful cravings? Stop nocturnal binging?* Or feel less inclined to eat bread? I've found that most people want to eliminate or limit specific foods or eat less. In

---

*In my experience, roughly one-third of my clients who are overweight eat in the middle of the night.

other words, most people want more control over when, what, and how much they eat.

As long as he or she is addressing a food habit, it doesn't matter if the person wants to change one relationship or twenty relationships with food. The process can be as targeted as Lay's potato chips or as general as cutting out all salty snack foods (which we specify). Once I am clear about the client's early messages and the habits that emerged, we will do a Release, letting go of these behaviors and introducing an Anchor Statement to the subconscious (I will do this with you in Chapter 6). An Anchor Statement is essentially a positive phrase—for example, "I control food. Food cannot control me"—that literally ties a person's subconscious mind to the conscious desire to be lean, strong, and healthy. The Anchor Statement is the linchpin of the entire process, as it is something you can use anywhere, anytime to curb craving, overeating, or binging (more on this in Chapter 6). Once we create an Anchor Statement and do a Release, I will help the client draw a new food blueprint—the client's dream relationship with food (I will do this with you in Chapters 7 and 8). And then I will ask the client if he or she feels ready to begin realizing this dream. I want to hear the client say in his or her own words, "Yes, I am ready to change." Once I'm convinced that the client is committed to the process and him- or herself, I begin the actual hypnosis session. This session lasts for about twenty minutes (I will guide you through this process in Chapter 9). The first five to seven minutes is just me talking, helping the client to become more relaxed so that he or she can experience the relaxed, focused alpha state and see that it can be brought on at will, anywhere and anytime it is desired. We will offer the subconscious mind a new picture using the words and images that describe the client's new dream picture of his or her relationship with food. When I'm finished talking, I ask the person to become more aware of his or her external surroundings, and we're done. This session is recorded onto a CD, which is given to the client. Once the session is done, I will instruct the client to listen to the CD every night while falling asleep until he or she meets with me for the second appointment, which is usually in ten days. As you probably have guessed, listening to the CD every night reinforces the new food blueprint that the client and I have drawn up in our first session.

You will learn in Chapter 4 that the formal name for repetitively talking to the subconscious mind in the alpha state is neurolinguistic programming (NLP). Dr. Milton Erickson, the father of hypnotherapy, used NLP with nearly all of his clients. Because we establish our unhealthy blueprints through the repetition of words and pictures and the associations between them, it makes sense to use the same approach to establish a healthy blueprint. NLP gives us the new healthy words, associations, and pictures. Repetition in the alpha state accelerates the absorption of the new picture. It's like the difference between a pencil drawing and a full-color oil painting. When it comes to the subconscious, the greater the impression and the more it's reinforced, the more powerful the impact. Neurolinguistic programming, which repeats the new picture using words and images, makes the new picture that hypnosis introduces stick. If clients use this first CD every night, most find that just the black-and-white outline of the first hypnosis session and a week of coloring in have radically changed their relationship with food.

A week to ten days later, the client comes in for the second session, which takes about half an hour. I will ask how things are going, what is working, and where there's resistance, if any. More often than not, the behaviors—snacking, craving, overeating, nocturnal binging—will have begun changing during the first week. Some people might find that one or two foods or habits still pull at them. There is an obvious reason for this: As with all computer connections, there are thicker and thinner wires. The thicker wires, carrying more charge, will be harder to sever, whereas the thinner wires will break more easily. For instance, if a person has a lifelong relationship with chocolate but can take or leave cheese, it may take just a day or two to reframe cheese, but more time for the call of Godiva to weaken.

In the second session, we create a new script based on the changes the client has experienced thus far, which will become the basis of the second hypnosis session (we will do this together in Chapter 10). Rather than suggesting that there is going to be a change, this second script acknowledges that there has been a change. It reinforces the subconscious mind's new, good food habits and gives the resistant old habits a kick in the pants. Like the first, this second session takes about twenty minutes. I also record this session, and the client leaves with the CD and instructions to listen to it every night for two weeks. Again, this NLP will bolster the new, healthy food blueprint and continue to weed out the key problem spots we identified in the second session.

At the end of the second session, I tell my client to have a State of the Union meeting with him- or herself in two weeks to assess progress. Does the person feel less attracted to unhealthy foods and less inclined to engage in unhealthy behaviors? Has the struggle with food lifted? Is the person making healthy choices? Is the person using food as fuel for health and well-being? Is the client in control of what he or she was not in control of before?

If the client is still experiencing resistance, I will see him or her for a third session. In some cases, there is a larger issue at hand, such as in the case, in Chapter 2, of John's fear of having an extramarital affair were he to lose weight. Roughly 80 percent of my clients don't have a confounding issue like John's and don't feel the need for a third session (Chapter 12 is devoted to troubleshooting issues and extending your success). After three weeks, most people feel in control of food rather than that food is in control of them. They are also usually amazed. In three weeks, they have effectively reprogrammed a lifelong challenge, and they can get on with the business of losing weight and living their lives. I tell these clients to continue to listen to the CD every other night until they reach their goal weight. They can listen every night, but every other is enough.

Generally, the amount of weight people lose per week depends upon how much they have to lose. A person who has to lose only 10 or 20 pounds will lose 1 to 2 pounds a week, which is the National Institutes of Health's recommendation for safe and healthy weight loss.[5] But I've also had morbidly obese clients lose 16 pounds in their first week. My favorite story, though, is one client who lost 13 pounds in her first week just by cutting Coca-Cola out of her daily intake!

Once people reach their goal weight, they enter the third phase of the Lite-State Method: Reinforcement. For those who want to stay at their goal weight for the rest of their lives, I recommend that they listen to the second CD once a week or once every two weeks for the rest of their lives. This is a way for them to check in and continue to reinforce their new food blueprint. As you know, I went through this entire process twenty-five years ago, and I still listen to my CD once every few weeks. Because of this, I have never fought to stay thin; I am simply healthy and fit. More often than not, if the client listens to the CD on a fairly regular basis, I will never see him or her again. But, about six months to a year later, I usually do hear from them. My clients write, call, e-mail, or fax to thank me, asking what they can do for me because I am the man who helped them save their marriages, their minds, and their lives.

One of the most powerful stories I can tell you is about a client whom I'll call Bob.

Bob's Story

Weighing roughly 800 pounds, Bob was in the category of super-morbidly obese.* In fact, he was so overweight that he had been trapped in his house for seven years because he couldn't fit through his front door. Bob's sister called me, asking me if I thought it was possible to use medical hypnosis to help him. They had tried everything, and she was afraid her brother was going to die. He had heart disease, diabetes, and severe circulation problems, and doctors and nurses were visiting regularly to monitor his condition. I had worked with a few super-morbidly obese people before, but none who was of Bob's size or severe condition. But I told his sister I thought medical hypnosis was worth a try.

I went to Bob's house. The entire house had been reconstructed—interior doors widened, floors bolstered, bathroom outfitted—to support his weight. I must confess that I was shocked by Bob's size. He was so big that he nearly covered an entire queen-size mattress. After some brief small talk, we got down to business and I asked Bob about his diet. His breakfast included twelve eggs, half a loaf of bread, a half pound of bacon, and a couple pints of orange juice. He went on to describe his

---

*A medical condition known as Prader-Willi syndrome can be the cause of morbid obesity. It is a genetic disorder involving the hypothalamus, the part of the brain that helps regulate, among other things, hunger and satiety. Everyone should have a medical evaluation prior to beginning any weight-loss program.

midmorning snack, late-morning snack, lunch, early-afternoon snack, late-afternoon snack, dinner, post-dinner dinner, midevening snack, late-night snack, and middle-of-the-night binges. Bob was eating round the clock, consuming about 15,000 calories a day. This man was doing everything he could to eat himself to death. I was overwhelmed and moved.

We talked about his history, and I asked him if he was ready to stop killing himself. He told me he was. Because he was so overweight, we came up with a new food blueprint that would make Bob attracted to lean proteins, vegetables, and water. Nothing else. Then I asked him to relax and find his alpha state. Once he was in a trance, the meditative state, I read the new blueprint to Bob and recorded it. I told him to listen to the tape while he fell asleep every night for a week.

A week later, I returned to Bob's house. He was amazed. His intake had dropped from 15,000 calories a day to 5,000. He was thrilled, and so was I. We did a second session, reinforcing the positive new behaviors and strengthening his aversion to unhealthy foods such as pastries, junk snacks, and soda. Again, I recorded the session and told him to listen to it every day for the next month. (I didn't want to take any chances, as his bad eating habits were so profound.) He lost roughly 40 pounds in the first month.

I continued to visit Bob at his home every few weeks for a year. In this first year, he lost 375 pounds, weighing in at roughly 425 pounds. As he progressed through the year, his caloric intake ultimately dropped to about 3,000 a day. After that, I saw him once a month for six months and he lost another 125 pounds. A year and a half later, in the spring of 2004, Bob emerged from his home. I was there. He walked out and put his arms up in a V, seeing the sky and the clouds for the first time in seven years. Today, while still overweight, Bob continues to lose. His life is not at risk, his diabetes is in check, he's on half the dose of blood pressure medicine he used to be, and not only can he walk to his bathroom, but he has the freedom to go anywhere he wants. After a lifetime of overeating, Bob eats like a normal, healthy human being.

The point of all this is to tell you that medical hypnosis is the most powerful tool for weight loss and weight control I know. It saved my life and has helped thousands of my clients to lose tons of weight and keep it off. But the best part about medical hypnosis is that you don't need to be a doctor or even a therapist to take advantage of this tool's healing power. You just need to follow the instructions in the remaining six chapters of this book and use medical hypnosis to draw a new food blueprint and create a new life in the privacy and comfort of your home.

The following methods and approaches that I will teach you will provide you with the exact same tools and information that you would get if you came to see me in person. Step by step, these chapters will hold your hand, challenge you, believe in your capacity to gain control over food and lose weight, and offer you a chance to have the healthy body and life you dream of.

Change Your Mind, Change Your Body

Chapter Four

Imagination is more important than knowledge.

—Dr. Albert Einstein

I f you're anything like 50 percent of my clients, you are probably skeptical about this whole "change your mind" process and wonder if it is really a viable approach to treating your weight issues. (The other 50 percent of my clients are referred to me by previous clients, psychologists, and physicians, so they are typically less skeptical.) Few people understand the true nature of medical hypnosis, and many regard it as a trick or parlor game, so questioning this approach is completely understandable. This chapter is devoted to explaining and proving the scientific validity of hypnosis and why it is so highly effective in addressing overeating and weight control.

A Balancing Act

Let's begin at the beginning: with your body. While you probably know most of the information that follows, it is important to remember that your body is made up of multiple systems that work together to keep you alive, healthy, and strong. The systems include:

- **A skeletal system,** which includes cartilage, tendons, ligaments, and 206 bones.

- **A muscular system,** which includes more than 600 muscles throughout the body.

- **A cardiovascular system,** which includes your heart, blood vessels, and blood. Your heart is a double pump, distributing oxygenated blood to the body and bringing oxygen-poor blood back to your lungs.

- **A respiratory system,** which includes your nose, trachea, larynx, and lungs. The lungs deliver oxygen to and remove carbon dioxide from your blood.

- **A digestive system,** which includes your mouth, esophagus, stomach, small and large intestines, gallbladder, and liver. While the stomach is the first place where food lands, it's actually your small intestine that breaks food down and delivers the valuable nutrients to your body. The large intestine holds all the waste from your small intestine and stomach before your body excretes it. The liver is your largest intestinal organ and helps the body cleanse itself of toxins. It also plays a large role in regulating the sugar levels in your body. This is why alcoholics and diabetics often have swollen livers—high levels of sugar overwhelm and damage this important organ.

- **A urinary system,** which includes your kidneys, bladder, and urethra. Your kidneys clean your blood, producing urine, and your bladder is the stretchy sac that stores the urine until you excrete it.

- **An endocrine system,** which includes your hypothalamus, pituitary, thyroid, pancreas, and adrenal glands. Your pancreas provides your body with digestive enzymes, helping it to digest food and control your blood's sugar levels. But most importantly, the endocrine system oversees the balance of the body. It regulates any and every imbalance that the body experiences.

- **An immune system,** consisting of several kinds of white blood cells, which is what your body uses to fight disease.

- **A reproductive system,** which, as you know, is what allows us to produce offspring.

- **A nervous system,** which includes your brain, spinal cord, and peripheral nerves. The brain makes up about 2 percent of your body's weight but uses 20 percent of the body's blood. Thanks to special cells called neurons, which carry electrical signals, your brain is what drives all of the other functions in the body. According to *The Photographic Atlas of the Body,* neuron communication between the body and the central nervous system (the brain) travels at speeds of up to 180 miles per hour. The authors write, "Each day the body makes more connections than all the world's telephone systems put together."[1]

As you can see, all of these systems work to keep your body healthy, strong, and alive by maintaining a balance: the right amount of oxygen, the right amount of sugar and salt, the right temperature, the release of toxins. This internal balance is called homeostasis. Homeostasis is your body's magnetic north, its ideal state. And your body is perpetually trying to work to achieve health and homeostasis all day, every day.

When we overwhelm our bodies with too much food—sugar, salt, fat, or even too many vegetables—the body's systems go into overdrive to help us get back into balance. Our systems cannot keep up, so we gain weight and, even worse, become fundamentally unhealthy. Our immune systems get beaten down and we feel generally awful. And when we don't feel well, the last thing we want to do is to make the effort to exercise or even cook ourselves a proper healthy meal. We're so tired and lethargic that we automatically reach for whatever foods are easiest and most familiar. It becomes a vicious cycle.

Fortunately, there is one part of the body that, while affected by these poor conditions, can work with us to change this unhealthy behavior and imbalance: the brain. If you change your brain, the rest will follow. I have had thousands of clients who, once they have a new relationship with food, not only lose weight but also reverse their diabetes, lower their blood pressure, reverse heart disease, and get themselves into excellent physical condition.

It's all in the mind....

The last twenty years have brought enormous advances in our understanding of the brain and how it functions. Thanks to brain mapping, which is the science of literally mapping out the brain's landscape, we know much more about where and how our brains are affected and changed by our thoughts and environment. For instance, we know that when a person is afraid, we see more blood flow and activity in a person's deep limbic system and amygdala, which are the areas of the brain related to emotion. We also know that when a chocolate addict even thinks about taking a bite of Lindt dark chocolate, there is more activity in the craving center of the brain. For our purpose of understanding the brain and its relationship to food, the key areas of the brain include:

- The deep limbic system
- The amygdala
- The basal ganglia
- The prefrontal cortex
- Broca's area
- The cingulate gyrus
- The temporal lobes

The deep limbic system is about the size of a large peach pit or walnut and is located near the center of the brain.[2] With the amygdala, a tiny powerhouse lodged inside it that generates fear and dread, the deep limbic system governs some of our most primal survival instincts. According to Dr. Daniel G. Amen, a medical doctor, neuroscientist, nationally recognized expert on the brain and behavior, and author of one of the bibles of neuroscience, *Change Your Brain, Change Your*

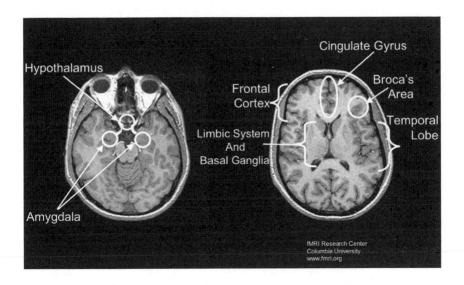

Life, the deep limbic system processes our sense of smell, moderates our libido, is responsible for our fight-or-flight response, controls our appetite and sleep cycles, stores highly charged memories (such as the death of a parent, abuse, or even being bullied by a classmate), and supports bonding with others.[3] Basically, without the deep limbic system, we would be robotic. And because of its role in processing smells and regulating appetite cycles, it is also directly linked to what and when we eat. In fact, in *Change Your Brain, Change Your Life,* Dr. Amen asserts that one of the key signs of imbalance in the deep limbic system is that a person's appetite is off.[4] In other words, the person is under- or overeating. In my opinion, because of its relationship to highly charged memories, the deep limbic system is also a key player in our emotional attachment to food and what it means to us.

According to Dr. Amen, the basal ganglia are a "set of large structures toward the center of the brain that surround the deep limbic system."[5] Dr. Amen and other internationally recognized experts, such as UCLA's Dr. Jeffrey M. Schwartz, agree that this area of the brain sets the body's "idle speed" or resting rate of activity.[6] This means that this is the part of the brain that tells us when we are hot, cold, emotionally comfortable or uncomfortable, anxious, scared, in lust, and in love. Overactive and underactive basal ganglia limit a person's ability to handle stressful situations. People who suffer from overactive basal ganglia usually experience heightened anxiety, have feelings of panic, and freeze when they should be acting. In contrast, a person in a stressful situation who has underactive basal ganglia feels flooded by the stressful stimulus and is compelled to act, but the person is completely unfocused and his or her actions do not address the stress.[7] Even if your basal ganglia are only mildly out of balance, it means that your sense of feeling comfortable in your own skin—physically, emotionally, and spiritually—is off. This means that you are going to seek out things that make you feel more at ease, more comfortable. And if eating makes you feel more comfortable, then of course that's what you're going to be inclined to do when you are stressed.

The prefrontal cortex sits right behind the forehead and accounts for about one-third of the brain. It is the most evolved system in the brain, governing our ability to learn, focus, plan, think critically, distinguish the real from the unreal, feel empathy, know right from wrong, and control our impulses.[8] Neuropsychiatrist Dr. Thomas Gualtieri describes the role of the prefrontal cortex as "the capacity to formulate goals, to make plans for their execution, to carry them out in an effective way, and to change course and improvise in the face of obstacles or failure, and to do so successfully, in the absence of external direction or structure. The capacity of the individual to generate goals and to achieve them is considered to be an essential aspect of a mature and effective personality. It is not a social convention or an artifact of culture. It is hardwired in the construction of the prefrontal cortex and its connections."[9] In other words, our prefrontal cortex is what defines our essential self and personality. But for our purposes, the most important aspect of the prefrontal cortex is that it can distinguish feelings from facts and right from wrong. So it enables us to know when we really are hungry and need food and when we are eating for other reasons. This is the part of us that talks to us when, after we've just had a satisfying meal, we find ourselves heading to the kitchen for a snack. The prefrontal cortex says, "I know I shouldn't be eating more, but . . ." Because of its ability to learn, use logic, and distinguish the real from the unreal, the prefrontal cortex is also the key to your ability to change your overeating patterns. It is what helps you know the difference between a feeling and a fact and the difference between a craving and true hunger. We capitalize on this ability when we use medical hypnosis. Broca's area is the section of the brain that involves language processing, speech production, and comprehension. It's named after Pierre Paul Broca, who discovered it in 1861, after conducting a post-mortem study on one of his speech-impaired patients. I mention Broca's area for this reason: The therapeutic use of hypnosis weighs heavily on language (in addition to imagery). You can see how damage to such a vital part of the brain would impact the success of hypnotic suggestion. Broca's area is just one example of the many aspects of the brain involved in verbal and nonverbal communication.

The cingulate gyrus runs longitudinally through the middle of the frontal lobes of the brain. The cingulate gyrus is what gives us the ability to shift our attention, to adapt to situations and ideas, to see things more than one way, and to cooperate with others.[10] A key indicator that someone's cingulate gyrus is out of balance is that the person seems stuck in one gear and has one cycling pattern of thought. In other words, the person is obsessed with something or someone. This manifests itself as having a rigid personality, chronic pain, road rage, argumentativeness, and addictions to alcohol, drugs (prescription or street), gambling, and food. The cingulate gyrus is extremely susceptible to stress—physical, emotional, and psychological. So this means that if you were or are stressed, particularly as a child, overeating might be one of your cingulate gyrus's responses to that stress. Fortunately, the cingulate gyrus is also extremely susceptible to stress relievers, such as reframing and meditation, which we will use to unlock your brain's ability to change its relationship with food.

The temporal lobes are located below your temples and behind the ears. You have a left and a right temporal lobe. The left side is usually dominant and processes language, retrieves memories and words, processes visual and auditory stimuli, and is associated with our ability to be emotionally stable. The right temporal lobe processes facial expressions and auditory stimuli, including voice tones, music, and rhythms.[11] We often talk about our "gut feelings," but our temporal lobes are what give us these gut feelings. For example, we instantly feel safe with a stranger on a bus because of his or her facial expression and body language. When explaining this to my clients, I often use the example of the way dogs sniff each other upon meeting. From that one experience, they intuitively know if they like or don't like each other. Our temporal lobes are just a more sophisticated system of this kind of intuition and judgment. So how do they relate to an eating imbalance? While they are not as directly connected to our eating as the deep limbic system, the prefrontal cortex, and the cingulate gyrus, the temporal lobes rule our mood. As you know, when we're in a particularly bad mood (think of the holidays) or an extremely good mood (think of the holidays), we're likely to eat more. The other very important thing about the temporal lobes is that their relationship with language is what makes changing your mind through medical hypnosis possible. The brain is the *only* programmable organ in the body, and it is programmed through words and images—but we will get to this in a moment.

As you know, merely telling ourselves to stop eating anything with sugar in it, or that we're not going to binge starting on Monday, or that we're not going to eat bread anymore, or that we're going to start exercising is not easy. If it were, we'd all eat only to fuel our minds and bodies and be incredibly fit and healthy. But, as we explored in Chapters 1 and 2, in our modern society of psychological eating, our brains are not programmed this way.

When we are young, our brain hardware—the deep limbic system, the amygdala, the basal ganglia, the prefrontal cortex, the cingulate gyrus, and the temporal lobes—is trained to trigger certain patterns. These patterns essentially are wirelike connections that are forged and fortified, becoming our software. In other words, as we grow up, we learn—from experience and watching others—how to respond and feel emotions about people, places, and things. The more we experience something, the more hardwired our response becomes. So if as children we learned that food is soothing or a way of relating, this will become part of our eating wiring. Fortunately, this wiring is plastic—it can change.

The Plastic Mind

I always talk to my clients about neuroplasticity because this is what makes change and human evolution possible. According to UCLA's Dr.

Jeffrey M. Schwartz, author of the landmark book on neuroplasticity *The Mind and the Brain*, "neuroplasticity refers to the ability of neurons to forge new connections, to blaze new paths through the cortex, even to assume new roles."[12] This means that your brain, my brain, anyone's brain—from eight to eighty—can be rewired (in the absence of certain degenerative brain diseases).

The idea of neuroplasticity was first developed when doctors realized that people who had suffered a stroke could relearn how to walk, write, or move their bodies. By definition, a stroke occurs when a part of the brain is denied oxygen or when a blood vessel in the brain bursts, sending blood into the space surrounding brain cells. Both events kill brain cells. People who suffer a stroke often feel dizzy, weak, and confused, have trouble seeing, lose their balance, feel numbness, or lose mobility, often on one side of the body. But what doctors and scientists have found is that even though the brain cells that are wired to tell the right side to move don't work, after time and with physical therapy, the person can learn to move that side of their body again using another part of the brain. This means that the brain is able to forge new pathways. The damaged part of the brain is circumvented—the rerouting makes this possible.

Another example of neuroplasticity can be seen in children who are born deaf. In *The Mind and the Brain*, Dr. Schwartz reports that scientists have found that in congenitally deaf children, the brain reassigns the children's auditory cortex (the part of the brain that normally processes what we hear) to process visual information instead.[13]

What makes a brain's neurons different from a kidney's or stomach's is the fact that the brain has what are called axons and dendrites. Dendrites are the parts of the brain's cells that look like tree branches or an octopus's arms. A dendrite's sole purpose is to look for electrical activity from other cells and carry that information to its cell. Likewise, an axon's sole purpose is to carry information out to other cells. As I mentioned earlier, this transfer of information happens at a speed of 180 miles per hour. Axons and dendrites are what allow the brain to make connections and forge new pathways. Dr. Schwartz writes, "Axons and dendrites enable neurons to wire up with a connectivity that computer designers can only fantasize about."[14]

According to the findings of Sara Lazar, Ph.D., of Harvard University and her fellow medical researchers at Massachusetts General Hospital, the more we use our brains, the more dendrites we grow. This is true regardless of our age. In fact, they have found evidence of more dendrites in active sixty-year-old men and women than in men and women in their twenties. They also found that the brain's cortex is thicker among those who meditate and exercise. This means you can strengthen and change your brain for the better![15]

Because we have the ability to make our brain stronger by making new connections, we can rewire our brain to change its habits—particularly self-destructive patterns such as overeating, craving, and thinking about food when there is no need to refuel. As I explained in Chapter 3, the Alpha Solution uses three steps to make these new connections:

1. Release—we formally let go of the old picture and messages.

2. Reframe—we provide our brain with a new picture.

3. Reinforce—we strengthen the new picture by repeatedly presenting it to the brain.

This simple three-step process works because our subconscious mind does not know the difference between fantasy and reality. In fact, the brain perceives fantasies and real experiences as the same thing. Don't believe me? Think about a nightmare you have had. Did you wake up with your heart racing? That's because your subconscious mind thought that whatever was happening in the dream was real. This is why a scary dream scares you and why you feel good when you wake up from a pleasant dream. Our reality is made up of a set of images that are presented to the mind again and again, making them recognizable and "real." If you presented your mind with a "reality" filled with healthy food preference and exercise over and over, then eventually that would be what is "real" to you.

So what are the implications of this plasticity? It means that the unhealthy patterns and pictures you have presented to your brain for years can be reimagined. You can present a new picture of yourself, the person you have consciously always longed to be—lean, strong, and healthy—to your subconscious mind, and your mind will believe it. We use the hypnotic or alpha state as a means of helping your mind release the old pictures and reframe and reinforce the new picture. We'll talk about how this works in the next few chapters, but all you need to know for now is that, thanks to neuroplasticity, we can change the unhealthy food blueprint to a healthy food blueprint in the brain.

The way we capitalize upon the brain's pliability is through the use of neurolinguistic programming. NLP involves the use of language to program the mind in the direction of one's choosing. Remember, the brain is programmable, and you have the code for this: words and your imagination. Medical hypnosis essentially introduces the idea of a change and a new picture to the subconscious mind. Neurolinguistic programming, which is essentially the repetition of the new picture using words and images, makes the new picture that hypnosis introduces stick. As I said in Chapter 3, medical hypnosis is the black-and-white outline and neurolinguistic programming is the coloring in. NLP essentially helps you live the picture you drew with hypnosis. In my method, clients listen to a customized CD every night for several weeks to color in their picture.

I use a CD because I feel it is the most effective means of capitalizing on the way we learn: through language and images. As you will see in later chapters, the languages and images you will be presenting to your brain are written by you and for you specifically. You will not be presenting any visions, pictures, words, or ideas to your brain that you don't believe in, approve of, or want.

Let me give you a practical example of how powerful the process of releasing, reframing, and reinforcing a picture with language can be.* A few years ago, I had the opportunity to work with one of tennis's rising stars. This guy was just an incredible athlete. He could hit a quarter anywhere on the opposite court seven out of ten times. He was ranked. He was on. He was it. But he had one big problem: his serve.

---

*I've found that while lawyers are some of my most doubtful clients initially, they respond to medical hypnosis exceptionally well. Because their lives are about finessing words, their brains are particularly trained to respond to language's nuance.

He could not serve faster than 130 miles per hour. And in the world of pro tennis, this was not enough for him. He wanted to be number one. After seeing every kind of physical therapist, massage therapist, trainer and coach, he came to me. It was his coach's idea. The tennis player thought the idea of medical hypnosis was ridiculous. Foolish. And he was scared that it might mess up his tennis mind. After much coercion and many assurances from therapists and coaches that medical hypnosis could do nothing but help him, he agreed to try it. After all, meditation, hypnosis, and guided imagery are cognitive techniques used by some of the world's elite pro athletes and Olympians.

As with all of my first sessions, we—the player, his coach, his therapist, his trainer, and me—sat down to discuss the problem. After they explained everything that he had done to improve his game and the kind of peak fitness he was in, I asked him to tell me what he said to himself as he got ready to serve. He said, "Well, when I throw the ball up into the air, I say, 'This ball is going to go like a chunk of metal to a magnet.'"

I asked him where he'd learned this phrase. He told me another coach had given it to him when he was a teen to help him with his accuracy. I said, "Obviously it has helped your accuracy, but think about what it has done to your speed."

Everyone in the room looked at me as if I were crazy. Then I said, "How fast can you hit a chunk of metal in the shape of a ball?" And then everyone in the room looked at me as if I were a genius.

I gave the tennis player a new metaphor to work with: a laser beam. Pinpoint, accurate, and *fast*.

I also made him a CD. I told him to not play tennis for a month and to work out and listen to the recording as he fell asleep instead. Again, they thought I was crazy. This tennis star had played every day for who knows how long. But I explained the idea of neurolinguistic programming to them and told them that his subconscious mind needed some time to draw the new picture and that playing would only call up the old picture, confusing his subconscious. Finally they agreed.

Eight days later, the tennis player called and said, "It didn't work."

I said, "It has not been thirty days. Do it for thirty days and then, if it doesn't work, we'll go from there." He laughed and we talked some more and I convinced him once again to try *not* playing and listening instead.

Eighteen days after that, twenty-six days after his session with me, he went out onto the tennis court and served a ball that went 137 miles per hour. And since then, he has gone on to have a tremendous career, consistently serving more than 130 miles per hour.

This is the power of neurolinguistic programming. This is the power of the human mind and your imagination. You *own* this potential. Everyone does! You can break through your glass ceiling!

The Stressed Mind

As you can see with the tennis star, we live in response to the messages we tell ourselves. For the tennis player, when he used his metal-to-magnet phrase, his brain responded one way. When he used the image of a laser, his brain responded in another way. I call this kind of interaction the mind-brain-body cascade.

The mind-brain-body cascade describes the flow of a thought, notion, or image, either real or imagined, from its inception (the first occurrence of it in the mind) into the brain (where it's processed) and the end result (the feeling or reaction it creates in the body) as "messaged" by means of the nervous system and chemical reactions. As I have said, by early adolescence each of us has a different brain program for how to respond to different events in the world. Our mother calls; we eat chocolate. Someone honks at us as we are crossing the street; we yell or jump out of the way or both. A person you have had your eye on suddenly kisses you; you blush. You watch your favorite TV show; suddenly the need to have pretzels or a soda pops into your head. This is the mind-brain-body cascade at work.

Believe it or not, all of these examples, including the kiss, are also stresses on the body. Because the body is constantly seeking homeostasis, it experiences outside stimuli as stressors—things that must be responded to. So if your body is trying to achieve balance after your boss has yelled at you and your partner has called crying, your mind and body are very stressed. They are using every tool they have to bring your body back into balance. And they would be stressed even if it were just one of these events. For many people, food-related behavior—overeating, snacking, and binging—is the number-one response to stress. This means the brain's neuropathways for stress have been "wired" to lead you to eat. But of course, this adds even more stress to the body, which is manically trying to restore the balance it craves and needs.

A few years ago, a doctor who was fifty-nine years old and the director of one of the world's most renowned medical centers arrived on my doorstep. He was more than 50 pounds overweight and was worried about diabetes. We did an inventory of his diet, as you will do in Chapter 5, and I found that his problem was just one food: bagels. He was eating as many as four a day.

Bagels have 20 grams of sugar in them, which can disrupt the body's liver and insulin functions, so his borderline diabetes was likely all due to his bagel habit. Beyond being sugar-laden, bagels are calorie-rich. At 350 calories a pop, the doctor was eating 1,400 calories a day just in bagels. I should also note that one 5-ounce bagel equals an entire day's Recommended Daily Allowance for bread and grains. Adding insult to injury, he typically ate those bagels with either cream cheese or butter on them. Imagine the calories now!

He told me that eating bagels had initially been his way of soothing his nerves (he was a stress eater), but now this soothing had become an obsession. He could not get through a day without eating them. He had tried everything, from Atkins to analysis, and nothing could curb his insane cravings for a bagel. Through analysis, he understood his bagel problem—the why—but could not change the behavior. And as a psychiatrist, he knew that diets were always a temporary fix. The doctor found me because he had recently read about the new research on neuroplasticity and that medical hypnosis was a credible method for harnessing the brain's neuroplastic ability. Coincidentally, he was trained in hypnotherapy during his residency. As he walked in, he said, "This is my last hope."

We talked about what he wanted. He also told me that he didn't want to have an aversion to bagels. He wanted to be able to occasionally eat a bagel and enjoy it, but to be more in control of the thought of a bagel. We did two sessions together, focusing exclusively on his bagel habit. In the first week, he dropped 8 pounds; he lost the remaining 45 pounds within nine months. His obsession was lifted along with the massive onslaught of sugar on his body, making his chance of becoming diabetic much slimmer. In fact, his blood glucose went from 110 to 92 within a month.

As we'll explore further in the next chapter, most people who struggle with food eat due to stress: early family stress, adolescent family stress, just plain family stress, work stress, relationship or lack-of-relationship stress, stress around food stress, weight stress, life stress. Well, guess what? Life is stressful. But what we have to remember is that it is our reaction to people, places, and things—rather than the things themselves—that shapes our experience. Stress is stressful enough on our bodies; our reactions to stress—such as eating—can hurt us even more. Fortunately, you can reprogram your body's response to stress using NLP to take advantage of neuroplasticity. And when you harness this ability with the Alpha Solution, you will achieve what your body has been looking for all along: balance.

A Place Settings

Chapter Five

> There was unanimous, automatic,
> unquestioned agreement around our table.
>
> —Winston Churchill

As I explained in Chapters 3 and 4, the first step of the Alpha Solution is to release the old pictures and unhealthy wiring. But before you can release your old patterns, you need to know what they are.

The first thing I ask clients to do is to describe their experience with food and eating as a child. It is essential to be aware of the early food messages because how we learn to eat as children is our blueprint for a lifetime of eating. The way our table was set—from the dishes to the food—establishes a lifetime of eating. I call these patterns place settings because it's not just what happened at the table. Our early interactions with food and eating determine how and when our neuropathways are formed and fortified.

In this chapter, we will explore and identify what food messages you were given, how your subconscious mind interpreted them and made patterns, and how these patterns have evolved into your current unhealthy eating habits. In Chapter 6, I will show you how to do a formal release where you will let these messages and patterns go. This release is the first step to changing your mind about food. But first let's look at food and your early relationship to it.

The Classic Place Settings

Food is our original and perhaps our most primal way (besides touch) of relating to and connecting with our parents. We are barely out of the womb and our mother is feeding us. It is one of our first interactions. As infants, we cry and we are fed. Over time, this builds a natural association between food and comfort. But this relationship can easily become skewed and the association overfortified. If the parent is using food as something other than nourishment to promote the baby's health and well-being—for instance, to quell the child's upset or irritability—then the association gets stronger. And if the parent continues to use food as a way to appease the child—a cracker or a cookie to calm a child making a scene in public—the association between food and comfort takes on kryptonite-type strength. We learn to crave dessert after dinner because that was the childhood reward for eating three more bites of chicken. We walk into the house and head for the kitchen because that is where the after-school snack was when we were children.

What was the dynamic between you, your parents, and food? Did your mother not feed you enough? Did your father deny you food if you misbehaved? Did your parents use food to quell your crying when they could not understand why you were upset and you could not talk to communicate your needs? If so, then it is no wonder you might still use food to make yourself feel better when you are upset. You have a primal association between food and feeling comforted. Did you get sweets as a reward for being good, doing your homework, helping with the dishes or trash, or not screaming in a restaurant? If so, of course you are going to treat yourself after you have worked hard or behaved in some heroic fashion. Your brain has been wired to associate being good or working hard with eating sugar. If you've ever said to yourself, "I'm going to have a slice of cheesecake as a reward after I lose 10 pounds," you know what I mean.

As we discussed in Chapter 4, early associations become hardwired and grow stronger as we get older. The more we repeat these behaviors, the more we reinforce our brain's neuropathways. That's why, these days, when you feel stressed or upset or bored or whatever your trigger is, eating feels like the most natural response. That's why when you binge you feel like something has taken over or possessed you. That's your brain's powerful patterning saying, "I know the route. I'll take it from here." For others it can be a smoke or a glass of scotch; the result is the same. A pattern is being reinforced and strengthened so that it produces an automatic conditioned response, which is just a fancy term for a reflex.

This is also why it is important to think positively. The more you think, "I cannot do this. I cannot be lean, strong, and healthy," the more the idea becomes hardwired in your brain and thus in your reality. Remember, it's all in your mind. Your thoughts (mind) dictate the response (brain), which in turn affects the body. As we discussed in Chapter 4, this is the mind-brain-body cascade at work. Everything starts with a thought; the cascade follows. Change your thoughts and you change the flow of the cascade.

So, what are your own patterns for eating? Shortly, I will discuss the most common early messages that generate the most common patterns of unhealthy eating. But as you learned in Chapter 4, the imagination is an extraordinarily powerful machine. What the early messages were can morph or evolve into amazing and unusual behaviors. My client Ron ate according to the fluctuations of the stock market (not uncommon in brokers and money managers). He would barely eat when the market was up and would binge when it crashed. Amy, a head copywriter at an ad agency, ate three to four heads of lettuce and mountains of carrots and other vegetables a day because when she was young her mother had told her this was great brain food. What her mother forgot to tell Amy was that any food, even vegetables, eaten in large quantities can be harmful to the body.

My point is that it does not matter how you eat now. Thanks to your Life Log and day-to-day experience, you already know how you binge, snack, overeat, and sneak food. You live with these rituals every day—

and probably have vowed to break them, if not every day, at least once a month. "I will not eat dessert tonight." "I will not have a second helping." "I will only eat half a bag." "I will not snack when I get home." "I will exercise and eat well tomorrow." "I'll diet on Monday." Yet you continue to do exactly what you so desperately try not to do. This is because you have a food blueprint (your subconscious mind) that was established early in your life and fights with your conscious desire to eat well and thrive.

So let us look at your history. What were the early messages that laid the foundation for today's unhealthy patterns?

Message #1: Crave crap.

Today, alarming numbers of us are raised on junk food. And even though these days you know that you should be eating healthy foods such as lean protein, complex carbohydrates, and green vegetables, you still crave the crap: fried fast food, soda, snacks with chemicals you can't even pronounce, candy that has five kinds of sugar and food coloring. If this is what you are used to, of course you crave the crap! Especially since it came from your mother or father, which makes the junk food even more powerful because it is associated with love, comfort, family, and compliance.

My client Bud is a great example of someone who had the patterning to crave crap. Bud grew up on fried chicken, collard greens loaded with chicken fat, mashed potatoes smothered with gravy, McDonald's, Hostess Cupcakes, candy, and donuts. As an adult, everything else tasted bad or "wrong." At thirty-one, Bud, who was a bus driver, came to me because he was concerned about his blooming waistline and high blood pressure. Once we identified his food pattern, I told him that the crave-the-crap food blueprint was actually the easiest message to address. All we had to do was reframe this message, teaching his brain to crave healthy, low-fat choices. It has been four years and Bud has lost 40 pounds. He has trained his taste buds and brain to choose foods that will promote his health and well-being, and he actually enjoys eating the healthy food more.

Message #2: Clean your plate.

There are thousands if not tens of thousands of members of the Clean Your Plate Club. As a child, they were told things like:

Clean your plate because people are starving in _____ [insert country].

Clean your plate or you will not get dessert.

Clean your plate or you will be on dish duty tonight.

Clean your plate or you will not get your allowance this week.

Clean your plate or you will not get to watch _____ [insert a favorite TV show].

Clean your plate or you will be punished.

A person who cleans their plate is a good person.

God only loves people who clean their plates. [This one is more common than you think.]

Waste not, want not.

Even more powerful are the parents who present this message from their own experience because they lived through periods of deprivation. This is not uncommon among Depression-era parents and grandparents, as well as people who survived the Holocaust or the pogroms, as in my father's case.

The biggest problem with these messages, beyond the fact that eating a full plate of food is generally not good for you (unless you are truly starving), is that cleaning today's plate is a much bigger challenge, because the plate is loaded with nearly double the calories it used to carry. According to a study done by the National Institutes of Health, twenty years ago the average hamburger was 333 calories; today the average hamburger is 590 calories. Twenty years ago an average serving was one cup of pasta with sauce and three small meatballs, totaling 500 calories; now it is two cups of pasta with three large meatballs totaling 1,023 calories. Twenty years ago a soda was 6.5 ounces and 85 calories; today the average soda is 20 ounces (roughly three times the size) and is 250 calories.[1] You get the idea.

Unfortunately, in our minds, a clean plate is a clean plate. So these days we are eating twice as much as we did twenty years ago, and a larger waistline is the result. The good news is that portion distortion is one of the easiest things to fix with medical hypnosis. We'll talk about how to change your mind's idea of what full means in the next few chapters, but for now, make a mental or written note that portion distortion is something you need to work on.

If you are feeling particularly guilty about leaving the food, put it in a Tupperware container and eat it tomorrow. If you are at a restaurant, get a doggie bag and eat the food tomorrow. If you are full and have not eaten everything on your plate, then that is okay. You are not a bad person. You are simply full.

Message #3: Have a snack as soon as you get home.

Do you walk from your front door straight to your refrigerator? Hundreds of clients tell me that there is a path worn from their front door to their kitchen. My client Carla described the daily experience as though the kitchen had a magnetic force. No matter what time of day or how full she was, Carla would walk into her house and feel pulled to her cupboards and fridge.

Growing up, Carla was a classic latchkey kid. She would walk home from school, do her homework, and hang out until her mother got home at around six or six-thirty. Carla's mother, trying to be a good mom, used to leave Carla surprise treats with notes that said things like "I'm sorry I'm not home" and "I love you even though I'm not there." So every day Carla would walk home, wondering what special cookie and note her mom had left for her. She would do her homework, watch television, and wait for her mom with the comfort of the food and note. But these well-meaning special treats and notes from her mom made a lasting and ultimately harmful association for Carla. She came to associate walking into the house with eating and feeling comforted. It was a love connection.

As she grew older, Carla would pick up other food on the way home to eat in addition to what her mother had left for her. And then she would be so full that she wouldn't eat much dinner. Her mother had no idea that the afternoon snacking had become a problem; she assumed that the extra 10 pounds Carla had gained was due to her build, or just adolescent weight that would eventually come off.

By the time Carla came to see me in her late thirties, she was 60 pounds overweight and was hiding her afternoon binges from her husband and children. As soon as she told me about the treats her mom used to leave her, I knew that her brain had been mapped for eating as soon as she walked into the house. Beyond doing a release—letting go of this old pattern and recognizing that it was harmful to her—we also looked at ways to keep Carla out of the kitchen. Currently it was her command center—she paid bills, made phone calls, and even kept her jewelry in the kitchen. Carla made a small space for an office nook in another room so that she had to walk to that room first when she came in the door to set her keys and mail down. The release along with this physical habit change completely changed Carla's relationship to the kitchen. She lost the desire to head straight to the fridge, lost 60 pounds within a year, and now knows that she can feel the warmth of her family as she walks in the door without a bag of cookies or a box of crackers.

So if your mother, father, or babysitter instilled the "have a snack as soon as you get home" routine, don't worry. The Alpha Solution—particularly the release—will do away with this habit once and for all.

Message #4: Want more.

Were you ever deprived of food as a child? Maybe it was not all foods, just the ones you wanted, such as sugary cereals or other junk food. Many people who suffered some sort of deprivation growing up—whether by circumstance or by punishment—emotionally and physically compensate by overeating as they get older.

The ironic thing about deprivation is this: It intensifies the longing for what you are being deprived of. You were not allowed to have dessert as a child, so now you want cake after every meal. Your parents sent you to bed without dinner, so now you eat enough for two every night to make up for those missed meals. This is the way deprivation works. And you will crave the food to the degree of your deprivation. It's like each time you eat you are saying, "I'll show you who is not deprived now!"

The other thing about deprivation is this: It makes you angry, and rightly so. It was and is unfair that you didn't get those meals, the dessert, the snack, the food you wanted and needed. So you go after whatever it was that you were deprived of with an enthusiasm and energy that can be forceful, aggressive, and eventually hurtful—to you.

Message #5: Eat as much as you can—for me (because I was deprived) and for the millions who were starved.

I have found that most people who were deprived of food or emotionally deprived produce a child who cleans the plate and becomes obese. Isn't it ironic how the generations can keep this fat cycle going? One generation who deprives produces an overeater who oversupplies his or her children with food, which produces another kind of overeater who will then deprive because they don't want their children to feel as overstuffed as they were. And on it goes . . .

This message of "eat as much as you can" is particularly true for children with parents or grandparents who survived a period of their life without food—a war, a famine, a concentration camp. As children, they hear this message at every meal.

My client Jeffrey's father was a Holocaust survivor who was starved in a camp in Poland for two years. Growing up, Jeffrey was relentlessly told by his father how the father had had to go without. His father had immigrated to the United States shortly after the war and determined his level of success by his big bank account and how heavy his children were. He literally wanted fat kids. Jeffrey told me that he used to say, "I want my kids fat and happy."

When Jeffrey arrived on my doorstep years later, he was 40 pounds overweight. Nearly the first thing out of Jeffrey's mouth was that he was feeling extraordinarily guilty about coming to see me. Even though his father had been dead for years, he said, "I can still feel him glaring at me if I don't finish what's on my plate. I can't imagine what he'd think of this—seeing someone to stop eating."

Jeffrey and I discussed what he was doing to his body and the fact that the fatter he got, the more severe the impact on his health. While his father had wanted him to be fat and happy, what he'd really wanted was for Jeffrey to be *healthy* and happy—only his torture had bound the idea of health and fat together. We did a release of the "eat as much as you can" message and then got to work on the unhealthy and deeply entrenched pattern of overeating Jeffrey had. Within six months Jeffrey lost most of the extra 40 pounds, and within a year he was at a healthy weight, exercising and free of his father's voice screaming, "Eat!"

Message #6: Food is love.

Your parents rewarded you with food. Instead of or even along with a pat on the back, you got ice cream or cake for an A or a home run. You broke your arm and got taken for ice cream. As with Carla, your mom or dad wasn't home much, so you got snacks or special meals as an apology and gesture that they cared. So these days, when you get a raise, win a case, or even when you lose weight, you reward yourself with a bowl of ice cream.

I don't think I've had a single client who has not described at least one important time in their life when food was offered as love. Valentine's Day chocolates. Birthday cake. Need I say more?

Remember, food is fuel for your health and well-being. It is not a connection to love or any other emotion. But used properly, food is energy that will allow you to give a hug, to go for a hike with a friend, to live so that you will feel love and connection.

While "food is love" is one of the most deeply entrenched and powerful wires in our brain, it too can be released and reframed. I will show you how in the next few chapters. For now, continue reading and looking for other potential patterns that need to be released.

Message #7: You must eat food made by relatives, close friends, and those in power no matter how full you are or how bad it is.

Your aunt Sue made the casserole. Your best friend (great person, terrible cook) brought cheese and bread to go with the meal you've cooked.

Your boss brings in cookies and you're on a diet. If something is offered, you eat it. No matter what, you serve it, eat it, smile, and say thank you, because that is what you were taught to do. It was all part of the good-manners program, because, according to your mother, father, or caregiver, if you didn't do these things you would be ungrateful or even selfish.

A few years ago two sisters came to see me. They were from a giant Italian family living in New York and, in keeping with tradition, every Sunday their mother hosted a big feast for the extended family. She was an exceptional cook, so bad food was not the problem. It was the amount of food they were expected to eat to show their appreciation— a seven-course meal, and all the courses were huge: antipasto; zuppa; insalata; primi (usually a huge plate of pasta); secondi (meat and fish) served with vegetables, bread, and risotto; cheese; and dessert. Their mother would say things like, "What do you mean, you're not going to eat it? I worked all week to get this meal on the table for you." The meal could last for three hours or more.

The girls were in their twenties and both were very conscious of their growing weight. As a result of these feasts, one sister was 25 pounds overweight and the other was closer to 50 pounds overweight. They would have been heavier if they had not taken precautions and measures to control their intake. Every Wednesday, they would begin a four-day fast to starve themselves so that they would be hungry and could eat the amount of food that was enough to please their mother. I told them that I was quite sure that, beyond these feasts, some of their weight gain also had to do with this starve/binge approach to eating, which can really harm a person's natural metabolic rate, slowing it down and causing more unnecessary weight gain.

Meanwhile, their mother was a rail-thin gym junkie, working out two hours a day four times a week. Essentially, the mother was giving her daughters all the food she was depriving herself of and dreamed of eating. The sisters told me that they had tried to talk to their mother but nothing had happened. They asked me to talk to her. I said I would do it, but only if the three of them came in together.

When the mother came in for the session, I allowed the sisters to share their experiences with their mother first. She listened. Then

I asked her if she would ever force-feed a child, shove food down its throat until it gagged. She looked at me with horror. "Never!"

I said, "Well, in essence, that is what you are doing to your daughters. You are forcing them to eat food they don't want."

The mother burst into tears and began apologizing. The three hugged, and that was the day all three of them began to draw new relationships with food. The girls had to learn to not feel guilty if they did not eat everything that was served. And their mother had to learn to eat what she needed so that she was not giving it to others.

Eating to please others is common, but it is not necessary. You do not have to do it to be liked, to be a good person or relative, or to be good. I will show you how to do a release for this, but in the meantime, give yourself permission to say, "No, thank you." And give yourself a pat on the back when you do.

Message #8: Don't even try to keep up with me.

Children of successful and/or very good-looking, thin, gym-going parents often get this message. Some people respond by becoming more successful, fit, and fabulous than their parents. Other people respond by becoming significantly less successful than their parents. One way to buck the parents' trend: retaliation eating. Over the years, I have had many clients who have told me that their unhealthy eating habits began out of spite. They knew that their parents would be upset and embarrassed by a fat child because it would reflect badly on the parent. And while it often is a successful way to get the attention and concern of a parent who is distracted by his or her success, the tragedy is that it is usually negative attention, which further damages the child. The child learns to get attention in an unhealthy way—by acting out rather than performing—and gains excess weight at an early age, which strains the body and leads to things such as early diabetes, high blood pressure, and heart disease.

My client Kristen was a classic example of a retaliation eater. Kristen was in her mid-teens when she came to see me. She was an only child, living in an extravagantly wealthy neighborhood just outside Manhattan. Her father worked eighteen hours a day as a banker and her mother was a phenomenally successful and beautiful psychologist, author, and professor. On the outside, everything looked great: big house, gorgeous and successful parents, excellent school, vacations in exotic locales. Kristen was the envy of many girls in her school. But inside, she was not happy. Her parents were so busy with their careers that they spent little or no time with her. And when they did, the parents were constantly coaching and correcting her. This resulted in her not feeling good enough for them.

Kristen's response was to give up trying to be as successful as her parents. Her first act was to dress poorly. This got her mother's attention, and she began to spend time on Kristen's wardrobe, trying to get her to wear dresses, skirts, and anything pink. Even though it felt like a corrective jerk, for Kristen the attention was delicious. So she tried to take it further. She began overeating, which again got her mother's attention. The only problem was that once she started eating, she found she could not stop. Then her mother's attention, which had felt good, felt bad. Comments like "You should be exercising more. The reason I have such a great figure now is that I started early" stung. So Kristen ate even more to soothe herself. The relationship between food and comfort was strengthened.

Finally, Kristen's parents sent her to a psychologist, which made her feel like more of a failure in their eyes. After a few short years, she was more than 100 pounds overweight. Kristen heard about me through a friend of a friend and came for help. I told her that she had to stop comparing herself to her mother and start living her life or she was going to kill herself. It had nothing to do with outside appearances; she had to respect her life, her process, and her talents.

Kristen heard me. We did a release and then made a CD to help her break her particular eating habits. She lost 75 pounds in the first year, and five years later does not feel the pull to compete with her mother.

Message #8A: Don't even try to keep up with them.

The don't-even-try-to-keep-up-with-your-siblings scenario is very similar to the successful, good-looking parent scenario. Among your siblings, you were the heavier child. It was so hard to compete with them because you felt you were not as athletic, smart, good-looking, and so on. So you went the other way, in the extreme. You gained weight as a way of *not* competing or of retaliating against your siblings' seeming perfection.

Two years ago, a young man named Max walked into my office. He was the younger brother of Margaret, the most beautiful and popular cheerleader in high school. Growing up, he would hear his sister and her friends talk about the hot guys at school with their six-pack abs and athletic achievements, and about how the girls had humiliated the occasional "loser fat boy" who tried to ask one of them out. Four years younger than Margaret and with some baby fat on his belly, Max feared that his high school years were destined to be filled with humiliation and teasing. So the summer before his freshman year, he tried exercising. Margaret thought this was funny. But, to his surprise, his parents were supportive of his endeavors. His mother thought Max might be a "late bloomer." After three miserable months of running, however, Max's belly remained. Throughout high school, Max tried many approaches—sit-ups and push-ups, dieting, laxatives, vomiting—but nothing ever worked, and he felt terrible. What was even worse was the realization that he would never have the superb definition of the guys his sister and her friends admired. With that, Max gave up and began eating. He told me he'd been 50 pounds overweight by the time he was twenty. And when he came to see me at 30 he had just been diagnosed with type II diabetes.

As with Kristen, we did a release where we let his comparative habits go and created a CD that reinforced the idea that he should walk his own path, becoming the best person he could be. In just a year, Max reversed his type II diabetes, got into excellent physical shape with an exercise program that worked for his body, and found a woman who loves him for who he is.

Message #9: Eat to protect yourself.

In my experience there are two common traits in people who use food to build armor around their bodies: those who have had injuries and/or surgeries that have changed their body shape so profoundly that they are embarrassed or ashamed of their appearance, and those who have been molested, abused, and/or raped and gain weight to protect themselves from other unwanted advances.

Faye had always been thin and healthy. In fact, when she came to see me she told me that she had never understood how people could be fat until she had breast cancer and had to have a double mastectomy. Then she understood. After her second surgery, she felt so uncomfortable, embarrassed by what she perceived as a deformed body, that she began eating bread and cheese to soothe herself. This attraction grew into an obsession, which gained her 60 pounds and a wall of protection. She said, "I didn't want my husband to touch me. So I made sure no man would look. A fat, breastless woman? Please. Can you think of anything more unattractive?"

I invited her husband in. He told me that her beauty had not changed in his eyes, and I could see that he was telling the truth. His love for Faye had not changed. I talked about what would make her feel better about her body. She said reconstructive plastic surgery. I said, "Let's do a release first. Let's let this undesirable image of yourself go so that when you have the surgery you really feel beautiful." Faye couldn't believe this was possible but went ahead and tried the release anyway, saying, "What more do I have to lose?"

We released the negative image she had of herself and Faye had an epiphany-like experience—she felt instant relief and love for herself. A few months later she had reconstructive surgery. And within six months she'd lost the weight she had put on, and was back in her life.

If you have gained weight as a kind of armor to protect yourself, especially as a response to severe trauma or abuse, I would strongly suggest that you seek out psychological counseling. This kind of patterning is fragile and should be handled with care because it is about your heart, which has been broken and needs serious attention, listening, and love.

Message #10: Eating relieves stress.

After twenty-five years of working with people who are suffering because of the eating patterns ingrained in their brains, I've realized that the blueprint of overeating that gets set in our subconscious minds early in life is all a response to one thing: stress. The stress of family life, the stress of school, the stress of feeling not pretty or handsome enough, the stress of not fitting in, the stress of too much attention or not enough, relationship stress, work stress, marriage stress, mother and father stress, the stress of getting older . . . I could go on.

The fact is that life is stressful. And, depending upon one's early life circumstances, people's subconscious minds learn to cope with this stress in different ways. Some learn to exercise, while others learn to starve themselves, drink, bite their nails, cut themselves, smoke, talk about it, sleep, or work it out. And many of us—particularly in the United States, where 66 percent of Americans are overweight—learn to eat.

My guess is that by now you have identified with one or more of the top ten messages. My greatest hope is that you are now aware of the external and internal forces that have precipitated your weight gain and that you now understand that these messages were planted early, watered and nourished as you were growing up, and then fortified and fed by eating. This has fueled your mind-brain-body cascade, solidified the neuropathways, and led you to where you are today.

What Are Your Place Settings?

In my office, after talking to clients about their histories and eating patterns, I go though a brief set of questions, called the Early Food Profile, to help them clarify what place settings they have at their food table. Likewise, it is time for you to make a record of your patterns.

You should answer these questions after reading this chapter and after at least a week of keeping your Life Log. As you answer these questions, go with your immediate, gut answer. Don't have a discussion with yourself or try to talk yourself into what you think is the right answer. The only wrong answer is a dishonest one, and that hurts only you.

Remember, the answers to these questions will provide key information for the release as well as the reframing portion of the Alpha Solution process.

Early Food Profile

1. When you are trying to diet, which do you find most difficult to do? *Rate these from 1 to 10, with 10 being the hardest.*

    * Control my portion sizes 10

    * Control my snacking   10

    * Control my cravings (by cravings I mean those times when a food comes to mind out of nowhere and you feel like you must have it immediately)   8

    * Denying myself what I really want   10

2. Do you eat due to stress or as a means of de-stressing?   10

3. Do you ever binge on food? (Forget about an academic definition of a binge. If you feel like you sometimes attack food or eat especially large portions, you binge.)   10 Chips

4. Do you ever purge food via extreme exercise, vomiting, or   1 laxatives? (If you are purging, I strongly suggest that you see a medical professional. Purging is common and extremely dangerous and can cause irreparable damage. If you continue, you can lose your teeth, get acid reflux, become malnourished, have a heart attack, even die. Yes, people do die from purging. So please, seek help.)

5. Do you ever eat in the middle of the night? (I don't mean late-night eating. This is getting up and eating in the middle of the night after you've gone to bed.)   1

6. Do you snack when there is no real need for food?   Lg

7. Growing up, were you ever told to clean your plate?   Lg

8. Growing up, was food ever used as a reward for being good?   Fries Lg Chips

9. Growing up, were you ever sent to bed without dinner?   Y

10. Do you use food in a way that is hurtful to you? This includes   Y overeating, binging, sneaking food, or eating extremely

unhealthy food. In other words, would you feed a child or a puppy or kitten the way you are feeding yourself?

Now, based on your answers to these ten questions, make a list of all the old messages and behaviors that you want to change your relationship with. This list is your Early Food Profile. When you are done making this list, ask yourself, "Am I ready to let these old messages and patterns go and commit to beginning a new path?" Finally, ask yourself one last question: "Do I really want this?"

If you are ready to smash the record that plays over and over and over in your head, then you are ready to do a Release, which is the first step in retraining your neuropathways to have a healthy wiring for eating. Read on to find out how.

An Important Note Before You Move On

You are about to begin the official three phases of the Alpha Solution process—the Release and then the first and second scripts (reframing and reinforcing). Until now you have been reading, reflecting, and learning about the method and yourself. This is a thoughtful, unrestricted process—in other words, you have been able to read and take action at your own pace. **Chapters 6 through 12 are time-sensitive.** As soon as you do your Release, you should move on to crafting and working with the first script and then, ten days later, the second. So before you begin to take this process on, make sure that you have time to do so. Remember, the more rigorously you apply yourself and give yourself over to the idea of change, the better the results.

Old messages:

1) You are too skinny — put some meat on your bones.

2) We'll stop for fries if you are good.

3) Keep out of the kitchen at night

4) Food provides comfort

5) Popcorn = happy family times together (Friday Night)

6) Go to bed without dinner if you are bad.

7) We don't have enough money for you to eat at the school cafeteria.

8) We don't have enough money to go out to dinner

9) Going to Thanksgiving or Christmas dinner means a day of boredom at nana's house.

10) Eat what is on your plate or you can't leave the table

11) Pizza is only for the adults

you need to have food to study

you don twant to go to bed hungry!

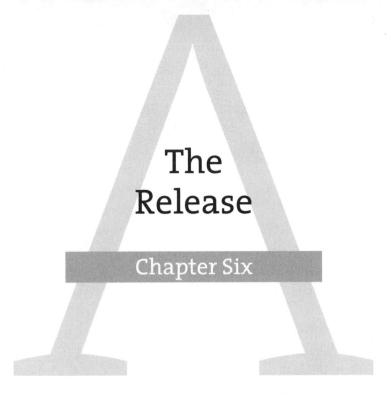

The Release

Chapter Six

Somehow, even before I heard the Buddhist teachings,
I knew that this was the spirit of true awakening.
It was all about letting go of everything.

—Pema Chödrön

Letting go of old patterns and early messages is perhaps the most profound step in the Alpha Solution. When we let go, we make space. When we let go, we invite and bring change.

What is a release? Simple. We make a formal statement to the subconscious mind that our old patterns of behavior—our tendency to snack each time we walk in the door, our use of food as a substitute for love, our weakness for chocolate—no longer exist. As we explored in Chapter 4, your brain cannot tell the difference between what it imagines and reality. Your thoughts—real or imagined—simply serve as software for the brain, and the brain sets the reaction in motion.

The formal release we use in the Alpha Solution relies on this same power of imagination. As I've explained in Chapters 3 and 4, in the release you will picture yourself putting all your old food patterns and messages in a huge box, sealing the box, shrinking the box, and then smashing the box to bits until it no longer exists. This essentially gives your brain the picture that these old messages no longer exist. It believes that what you pictured really happened and that those patterns have been obliterated.

You're probably thinking, "How could something as simple as using my imagination to picture myself putting my food struggles and unhealthy patterns in a box and smashing it really do anything? How could this be more effective than talk therapy? How could this possibly work?"

Well, first, when you do the Release you will be capitalizing on the brain's alpha state. You will be talking directly to your subconscious mind—the place where all the early messaging is stored, and the place that cannot distinguish between imagining lemon juice on your tongue and lemon juice actually on your tongue.

Second, while I believe that talk therapy can be extremely beneficial in many cases, I also know that by talking about these patterns and messages, we are keeping them alive. As wonderful as talking about a problem is—it often does lead to understanding—it also makes the issue even more of a reality. The problem can grow instead of subsiding. Whereas with the Release, we are literally telling the subconscious mind that the problem and patterns cease to exist. They are dead. End of story. End of the patterns.

Still don't believe me? Let's try it and see.

How to Do a Release

Doing a Release is perhaps the most important part of the process you have begun. Telling the subconscious mind that the struggle is in the past not only creates a parking space for the new desired healthy relationship with food but is also a major action and physical demonstration of your commitment to heal. It means you are on your way to taking responsibility for your mind and body.

When doing a Release, you'll need to make some time for yourself and the process. For the release to be truly effective, it needs to be done with the proper intention and integrity. In other words, what you put into it is what you will get out of it.

The first thing you need to do to get ready for your Release is to compose an Anchor Statement.

The Anchor Statement

As I mentioned in Chapter 3, an Anchor Statement is a short, empowering phrase that supports your desire to be lean, strong, and healthy. The most common Anchor Statement my clients use is "I control food. Food cannot control me."

This Anchor Statement will be used in all three phases of the Alpha Solution—releasing, reframing, and reinforcing. It is the key phrase in both of the medical hypnosis scripts you will be using. The phrase will become linked in both your subconscious and conscious minds to the process of healing. After using your Anchor Statement in the release, whenever you say the phrase to yourself, it will connect you to the release and your desire to be lean, strong, and healthy. Think of it as a touchstone that connects you directly to your desire to be well. You will find that once you start using it—when you have a craving, feel emotional, and want to binge or overeat—it will rescue you by anchoring you to your true desire to be lean, strong, and healthy. You can say it to yourself before eating a meal, at the movies on Saturday night, or at the office when the pastries arrive. After some time, you will find that saying the phrase also becomes an automatic message of relaxation, as it connects your mind to the relaxation and freedom you will feel after the release.

So, what is your Anchor Statement?

As I said, most of my clients use the Anchor Statement "I control food. Food cannot control me." But if this phrase bothers you or doesn't feel like your voice, you can write another empowering phrase and use that as your Anchor Statement. Here are a few examples.

- *I am free, now and forever.* [As with the popular "I control food. Food cannot control me" Anchor, this is good for those who struggle with cravings and the feeling that food overwhelms them.]

- *I am lean, strong, and healthy.* [This is good for those who are pulled by others—old parental messages, the need to clean their plate, others' influences—and need to connect with their truest desire and self.]

- *My body is precious and I treat it accordingly.* [This is good for those who overeat, binge, eat mostly junk food, or attack their bodies with food.]

achieving what I want and being with my family.

- *I value my brain, body, and life.* [This is good for those who fight stress, don't value their own worth (those who heard the "don't even try to keep up with me" message), and those who have suffered from trauma (cancer, abuse) and don't feel comfortable in their bodies as a result.]

You want to find a phrase that you can carry around and say to yourself on a regular basis. Most important, it should feel empowering. Try a few. Walk around with the statement you choose for a few days and see if it feels right. You can even combine phrases: "I am lean, strong, and healthy, and I am free now and forever." Make sure you connect with it. Above all else, make sure it inspires you.

Once you have an Anchor Statement you love, you are ready to do your formal release.

Let Go

Once you have an Early Food Profile (from Chapter 5) and your Anchor Statement, plan a time—at least an hour—and find a place where you can be alone, in a quiet space (no children screaming downstairs or television in the other room), and in a completely comfortable and supported position. This might mean sitting in a big lounge chair or lying on your bed or the floor, whatever suits your body.

To prepare for the release, follow these directions:

1. Read through the release script once.

2. Note that the first section of the release includes what is called an induction. As you will read, this induction is nothing more than a series of exercises where you tighten and release the muscles in your body. An induction is just a formalized way of helping you become relaxed and at ease. You will also be

using this induction method to relax in the two medical hypnosis scripts.

3. On your first reading of the release script, you will find places where I ask you to include your Early Food Profile and places where I ask you to include your Anchor Statement. Write them in.

4. Next, read through your personalized release script about four or five times. **Don't be concerned about memorizing this script word for word.** The process is more about picturing and thinking of yourself doing something than the language of doing it. In other words, use this script as a loose scenario and tailor it to fit your needs and imagination.

5. Once you feel comfortable with the script and have your Anchor Statement and Early Food Profile written in, make sure you are in a perfectly quiet space and have at least thirty minutes. Do whatever you need to do to make the space comfortable. Make sure that the temperature is right. You don't want to be too hot or too cold while doing the release, as it will distract you. Have low or soft lighting—no overhead fluorescent lights.

6. Once you have time and a calm and soothing space, find a position that is truly comfortable. Sit or lie there for a few moments and ask yourself if your entire body feels supported. If you become aware of a foot dangling or a shoulder feeling awkward, listen to this and adjust yourself until you are really and truly supported. Take your time. There is no rush.

7. When you feel relaxed and supported, close your eyes, breathe, and begin your release when you are ready. The actual release should take about twenty minutes.

The Release Script

Be sure you're in a comfortable position.

With your eyes closed.

The head and neck supported well.

Place one hand on your lower belly and feel it rising and falling as you breathe.*

Breathing in this way always helps induce relaxation and sleep.

Take a deep cleansing breath in through your nostrils.

And then a nice slow exhale through your mouth.

Just notice your hand rising and falling with each breath, indicating your belly is doing the work.

Take another deep cleansing breath in through your nostrils.

And a nice slow exhale through your mouth.

And repeat that one more time.

Inhale.

Exhale.

And when you complete this deep breath, continue to breathe in a normal fashion.

Through your nostrils.

If you have trouble breathing through your nostrils, then just breathe through your mouth.

And just continue to breathe normally.

Observe the flow of air coming in and out.

Try to leave the rest of the world on hold.

To help relax further:

Tense up all the muscles in your forehead.

Squeeze your eyes shut so they're squinched up as tightly closed as possible.

---

*The reason for doing this is to be sure that you are breathing from your belly. Your chest shouldn't be rising, nor your shoulders. Just the lower abdomen. Feel the belly rising and falling. Your chest and shoulders should be relaxed and at ease.

Clench your teeth tightly.

Now tense up all the facial muscles.

Tighten them.

Hold that.

A little tighter.

Tighter.

Tighter.

And relax, letting your facial muscles go.

Breathe.

Inhale.

Exhale.

Good.

Notice how good the facial muscles feel, so relaxed.

Now, be sure your head is supported well. No strain on your neck or back.

Let your head just feel heavy, supported, tension-free, easy.

Now, raise your shoulders toward your ears as if you're trying to touch your earlobes.

Higher.

Higher.

Higher.

And let them drop, like they have weights pressing on them.

Nice and heavy and relaxed.

Let them go.

Inhale.

Exhale.

Good.

Now, I want you to think of yourself as being as relaxed as a rag doll.

In fact, use that image.

Imagine you're looking at a rag doll just slumped in a chair.

Totally effortless.

Completely relaxed.

Imagine being that comfortable and relaxed.

Hold that image and thought in your mind as you continue to relax further.

Now tense up all the muscles in your arms.

Make fists.

Squeeze.

Tighter.

Tighter.

Tighter.

And release.

Relax.

Let those arms just drop and relax, like heavy weights.

Let them feel heavy.

Now bear down on the belly.

Tighten up your abdominal muscles.

Squeezing.

Tighter.

Tighter.

Tighter.

And relax.

Take a deep breath in through your nose.

And a nice long exhale through your mouth.

Let go of any remaining tension.

Drift and relax.

And finally, tense up all the muscles in your legs, from the buttocks all the way to the toes.

Flex your thighs.

Tense your calves.

Point your toes.

Hold that.

Tighter.

Tighter.

Tighter.

And let them drop.

Nice and heavy.

Like logs.

And relax.

Take another deep breath in through your nostrils.

And exhale, letting the breath out through your mouth, nice and slow.

Let it all go.

Notice how the body feels now.

How relaxed.

Like a rag doll.

Notice how slow your breathing has become and how much slower it will be over the next few minutes. Notice how cool the air is on your inhale and how warm it is when you exhale.

Good.

At this point, the body has moved into a meditative, profoundly relaxed state and will continue to do so with each breath.

Imagine now that you're in a very large room. A room the size of a ballroom.

You're the only person there.

And the only object in the room is a huge box sitting on the floor.

Make sure you see the box so tall that you have to look up to see the top. Picture it so wide that you can't see around it or get around it. And because it's so huge it must be heavy, and therefore too heavy to push out of the way.

Make sure you see the box as vividly as possible. It's a giant wooden cube. Give it a color. Give it a texture. Whatever allows you to see it with greater distinction.

Now put all the messages that you want to get rid of, eradicate forever, in the box. [This is where you include your early food profile material.]

Picture yourself lugging these heavy messages in a bag across the floor, dragging them up a ladder, and heaving them into the box.

Hear the thud as they hit the bottom of the box.

Now picture yourself sealing the box. Making it airtight.

Wrap it in a huge sheet of plastic.

Seal it up.

Now see that this box is completely sealed. It's airtight. Whatever is in it cannot get out.

These messages are sealed in the box.

And what is in that box is your old relationship with food. Your struggle. The messages you no longer require.

Think of everything in that box as being compartmentalized. Separate from you. Not part of you in any way. Disconnected from you and your life.

I want you to use your inner voice now.

Repeat each of the following phrases exactly like this.

Say the following phrase to yourself:

My craving for crap exists sealed in the box.

My need to clean my plate exists sealed in the box.

My need to eat as soon as I walk in the door exists sealed in the box.

The feeling of being deprived of food or love exists sealed in the box.

My need to eat as much as I can exists sealed in the box.

My need to eat to please exists sealed in the box.

My need to retaliate by eating exists sealed in the box.

My use of weight as armor exists sealed in the box.

My use of food to relieve stress exists sealed in the box.

See that everything in the box is in its rightful place.

Know that you cannot miss what you no longer want.

Say to yourself:

My conscious desire to be free of the struggle is represented by the box.

See how the conscious desire to be lean, strong, and healthy is now also the subconscious desire. The minds are synchronized now. They both want you to be lean, strong, and healthy without feeling deprived, without dieting—in fact, feeling empowered.

Say to yourself:

I am ready to take total control of my relationship with food.

Now I want you to imagine the box truly looming over you.

You're seeing it, you're looking up at it. It's towering over you.

It's a roadblock. And you need to get past it because on the other side is a door to health and well-being.

So you need to put the box in its proper place and perspective.

Now imagine that the box begins to shrink. Picture it getting smaller and smaller and smaller.

Still remaining sealed. Airtight.

Picture it now where it has become so small that you are looming over the box.

And picture it shrinking even further until it becomes the size of your thumbnail.

And picture it shrinking even further until it becomes the size of your pinky nail.

Now take a good look at your relationship with that box.

How can something this small have any control over you?

It can't. It's powerless. You can kick it, walk over it or around it, do anything you want to it.

It is in no way, shape, or form a roadblock to you anymore. You can see beyond it.

Not only did you take control of the box, but you've also changed your entire perspective on it. You tower over it.

The box is in its proper place. You have released your old food messages.

Rather than just feel in control of that box, now take this experience to the next logical level and picture yourself lean, strong, and healthy, crushing that box under your foot. Smash it down. Pulverize it. Feel and see how good that feels.

Feel the release of the struggle and the empowering feeling of being in control of food. Turn that struggle into dust.

You now control it.

You have eliminated it.

And as you do that, repeat this phrase in your inner voice: "_____." [Use your Anchor Statement here. You can use the phrase, "I control food. Food cannot control me." Or write an empowering phrase that works for you.]

When you're done crushing the box, picture yourself stepping back and looking down at what is left. It's nothing but dust.

The phrase "_____" [Use your Anchor Statement here.] *will forever be associated with the elimination of that struggle.*

The struggle is gone.

Anytime you use the phrase "_____" [Use your Anchor Statement here.] you are reminding the subconscious mind that you are in control of what, when, where, why, and how much you eat.

The phrase becomes a conditioned response, an automatic reflex to make a healthy choice for mind and body. This picture of the dust matches your conscious desire to be free of the struggle and to be lean, strong, and healthy.

So, in essence, your conscious and subconscious mind are in agreement. You are free of ambivalence. Conscious desire is your subconscious response. The phrase becomes more meaningful the more you use it; like any conditioned response (reflex), it becomes more and more automatic.

When you are done with the release, you should feel incredibly proud of yourself. Congratulations! To celebrate, you might want to burn your list of old messages and patterns. The struggle is in the past. Over. You have erased it. You have taken a giant leap. How do you feel? Relaxed? Lighter? Freer? You should.

Now that you have released your old messages, it's time to release and let go of the food itself. Onward!

If you cannot feel a difference right away or don't think the release did anything, don't worry. The most important action for now is putting that Anchor Statement, "I control food. Food cannot control me" (or whatever phrase you used), to use and reinforcing the meaning it has to your subconscious mind. **I want you to say your Anchor Statement to yourself *throughout the day*.*** Say it if you have a craving. Say it if someone brings a platter of cookies into the office. Say it when you pick up the menu in a restaurant. **Say it as you begin each meal.** Write it down and look at it throughout the day. Make it your screen saver. Stick it to the mirror in the bathroom or on the dashboard of your car. Do whatever it takes to cement this phrase and its power in your mind.

Now let's move on to Chapter 7 and begin the process of thinking about how you are going to reframe your brain.

---

*You can say the Anchor Statement out loud or use your inner voice. The result is the same.

The Alpha Solution Inventory

Chapter Seven

What is patriotism but the love of
good things we ate in our childhood?

—Lin Yutang

Once my clients release their old patterns, we can begin to dive into the process of looking at the foods and behaviors that feed their neuropathways for unhealthy eating. To accomplish this, I do an inventory with all my clients that helps us identify, assess, and describe their current relationship with food. In this chapter, I will guide you through the same process.

This chapter presents a series of lists, drawn from your experience and the Life Log you have been keeping, that will provide a comprehensive picture of what, when, and where you eat. This picture will then help you identify your relationships with particular foods and help you define the foods you want to have more control over and less desire for.

The first list is essentially a large grocery list. Go through it and mark the foods that have a particular draw for you. These are your "gotta have it" foods. For instance, does the mere idea of peanuts send you to the store for a jar of Planter's? Or are your favorite cookies something you would drive twenty miles to buy if you didn't have them in the house? If so, then you would put both nuts and the cookies on the "gotta have it" list.

Beyond identifying the "gotta have it" foods versus the "take it or leave it" foods, the reason I put my clients through this process is to demonstrate that not all foods are your problem. Let me say that again: **Not all foods are your problem.** In fact, there are probably only five or six foods—what I call a person's "staples"—that are responsible for your weight. Remember the Connecticut woman in Chapter 1 who was only 5 pounds overweight but struggling? It was just one food, watermelon, standing in her way of excellent health and happiness.

There is a significantly different brain pattern for the foods that pull at you and the foods that don't. For many of my clients, understanding that *all* foods are not the problem is a profound realization. It means that the task of retraining their brain is not nearly as huge as they thought. They don't have to teach their brains how to eat every food— just a few. This is also true for you.

The "take it or leave it" list also illustrates the goal relationship you want to have with the "gotta have it" foods. Soon, through using medical hypnosis and NLP, you will feel indifferent to foods that once sent you into a binging spiral.

The second phase of this inventory involves identifying where and how you are eating these foods. Again, as with your Life Log, this process is not designed to shame or embarrass you. It is to help you write a precise script that will weed out these behaviors and help you realize your freedom from food.

Now, let's get to work.

The Inventory in Action

The first thing I want you to do is go through the following list and write a **G**, for "gotta have it," next to any food that you eat in large portions, binge on, snack on, eat during the night, or just feel a great passion for. Mark an **I** next to all the foods that you feel *indifferent* about or could take or leave no matter what kind of binge you are on. And write a **B** next to those foods that feel *borderline*—you might binge on a B food if a G food is not around, but otherwise, it is not really an issue.

The list of foods I've provided to help you define your current food blueprint is as comprehensive as possible, but of course I can only go so far. For example, by my last count, there were twenty-seven different varieties of potato chips on the shelf at my local supermarket. A list of each and every food available would be a book in and of itself. This list is to be used as a guide to inspire and get you thinking, helping you draw the clearest, most precise picture of what you eat. This means two things. First, if I have written down potato chips, specify, along with the G, I, or B notation, what brand and flavor you prefer. For instance, if potato chips is one of your "gotta have it" foods, you'll want to note:

Potato chips **G** *Pringles Salt and Vinegar*

Second, if there is something not on this list that is a "gotta have it" food for you, add it to your list. Remember, the more specific you are now, the more specific and thus the more effective your script will be.

I recommend that you write directly in this book in the space I've provided. But if you don't feel comfortable writing in a book or have borrowed it from a friend or the library, photocopy these pages so that you can write on them. It is important for you to have a record that you can see. What you say to yourself and can remember will not be enough.

One final thought before you begin: As you go through and mark up these pages, go with your first, gut response. Don't have a discussion with yourself about each food. If you read "brownies" and your immediate response is "Yes!" include them on your "gotta have it" list. Or if the food is not your first-response-to-stress food but you do find that on occasion you will binge on that particular food, include it on the "gotta have it" list. For instance, when I did this twenty-odd years ago, my therapist said "pizza" to me, and I said, "Yes. Gotta have it." Even though I preferred peanut butter as a binge food, I knew that if I was in a situation where peanut butter was not around and pizza was, I could and would eat an entire pie.

Ready? Let's go.

The Inventory, Part I

Beverages

Water—mineral water, tap water, soda water

Coffee—this includes lattes, cappuccinos, and any other (often high-calorie) complex coffee confection you can get in today's coffee bars

Tea—caffeinated, decaf

Chai

Hot water with lemon

Orange juice

Apple juice

Cranberry or some combination of cranberry and other fruit juice

Grapefruit juice

Grape juice

Pear juice

Peach juice

Pineapple juice

Pomegranate juice

Apple cider

Milk—whole, 2%, 1%, nonfat, chocolate, vanilla, strawberry, coffee, cream on the top

Half-and-half

Cream—heavy, whipping, light (either liquid or whipped)

Soy milk—regular, low-fat, vanilla, chocolate

Rice milk—regular, low-fat, vanilla, chocolate

Oat milk

Almond milk

Root beer

Ginger beer

Ginger ale

Diet soda—Diet Coke, Diet Pepsi, Diet 7-Up, Tab, Fresca, etc.

Regular soda—Coke, Pepsi, Vanilla Coke, Pepsi One, 7-Up, Sprite, Mountain Dew, cherry soda

Highly caffeinated drinks such as Red Bull

Alcoholic beverages such as beer (in the bottle, from a can, draft), wine (red, white, rosé, champagne), and hard liquor (vodka, whiskey, rum, bourbon, gin)

Condiments

Mayonnaise

Mustard

Ketchup

Salad dressing—French, Russian, ranch, blue cheese, vinaigrette

Salsa

Nutella

Marshmallow Fluff

Jams and jellies

Peanut butter

Honey

Molasses

Brown rice syrup

Maple syrup

Brown sugar

White sugar

Powdered sugar

Dairy

Butter

Margarine

Sour cream

G Cheese—American, Cheddar, Brie, chèvre, Swiss, blue, feta, soft, firm, mozzarella, provolone, Parmesan, light and soy, Gouda, stinky, sheep's-milk, semisoft, by the slice, by the pound

Cream cheese

Cottage cheese

Mascarpone

Ricotta

Yogurt

Frozen yogurt—by the pint, in a bowl, in a cone

Ice cream—out of the container, in a mug, with a spoon, sundaes, cones

Bread

White

Rye

Sourdough

Baguettes

Rolls

Pumpernickel

Scones

Homemade

Cheap

Sliced

Used for cleaning the plate

With everything

Plain

Fruit

Apples

Bananas

Citrus (oranges, grapefruit, limes)

Grapes

Pears

Melons

Berries and cherries

Stone fruit (peaches, plums, nectarines)

Dried fruit (dried apples, dried apricots, raisins)

Pineapple

Mangoes

Salty, crunchy snacks

ᔕ Corn chips

ᔕ Potato chips

ᔕ Pretzels

Terra chips

ᔕ Cheetos

ᔕ Crackers

ᔕ Soy crisps

ᔥ Popcorn

Snack mixes

ᔕ Goldfish

Bread sticks

Lavash

Matzoh

Doritos

Fritos

Bagel chips

Nuts—peanuts, cashews, almonds, macadamia nuts, hazelnuts, pistachios, salted, honey-roasted, chocolate-covered

Sweet snacks and dessert foods

Brownies, blondies

Cookies—animal crackers, butter cookies, biscotti, chocolate, chocolate chip, diet-friendly cookies (ha! not when you are eating a box or two), Fig Newtons, fruit, ginger, graham, kosher, ladyfingers, nut, coconut, oatmeal, plain, rugelach, sandwich, wafer, cookie dough

Cereal—Cocoa Krispies, Cap'n Crunch, Frosted Flakes

Cakes—cheesecake, chocolate cake, pound cake, layer cake, tea cake, babka, cupcakes, store-bought, frozen

Pop-Tarts

Granola—bars or by the bag

Frosting—with or without the cake

Pie—apple, blueberry, peach, rhubarb, strawberry-rhubarb

Tarts—apple, berry, pear

Pudding—chocolate, vanilla, rice, bread

Soufflés—chocolate, pumpkin, cheese

Chocolate—white, dark, milk, with nuts, with fruit, plain, melted, chips, bars, bags, with espresso beans

Candy—hard, soft, chewy

The Inventory, Part II: What's Cooking?

Now, let's look at your pantry in terms of meals. Once again, go through the following list and identify the following meals as "gotta have it," "borderline," or "indifferent."

Breakfast foods

Eggs—scrambled, fried, over easy, sunny-side up, omelets, baked, poached, frittata, quiche

Toast—plain, with butter, jam, butter and jam, peanut butter, almond butter, apple butter, cheese

French toast—plain, with maple syrup, with maple syrup and butter, with strawberries, with whipped cream

Pancakes—plain, banana, chocolate chip, with maple syrup and butter, one, two, three?

Crepes—sweet or savory

Cereal—hot, cold, cooked, with milk, out of the box, in the afternoon, sugary, all-natural, granola, Grandma's special recipe, grits

Breakfast meats—sausages, bacon

Home fries/roasted potatoes—with or without cheese, gravy, hollandaise, fresh herbs

Muffins—blueberry, corn, blueberry corn, apple, banana, bran, small, large

Bagels—frozen, fresh, toasted, untoasted, loaded, plain, with cream cheese, lox, and red onion

Pastries—croissants, Danish, fritters, breakfast tarts, turnovers

Breads—banana bread, zucchini bread, carrot cake/bread

Donuts—any and every imaginable kind

Lunch foods

Cold cuts—salami, pastrami, turkey, roast beef, deli platters, antipasto plates

Chicken salad

Tuna salad

Lobster salad

Crab salad

Seafood salad

Egg salad

Pasta salad

Potato salad

Bean salad

Whole-grain salads—tabouli, wild rice

Coleslaw

Hummus

Baba ghanoush

Hot dogs—with sauerkraut, with chili, with ketchup

Hamburgers—with cheese, with cheese and bacon, loaded

Turkey burgers

Veggie burgers

Grilled cheese, tuna melts, reubens

Sandwiches, hoagies, subs

French fries

Onion rings

Dinner foods

Pasta—macaroni, fusilli, spaghetti, vermicelli, lasagna, rotini, farfalle, orecchiette, orzo, elbows, penne, rigatoni, ziti, angel hair, cannelloni, stuffed shells, macaroni and cheese

Pasta sauce—marinara, pesto, cream, meat

Pizza—gourmet, delivered, the whole pie, five slices, extra sauce, extra cheese, every way

Fish—fried, broiled, steamed, poached

Shellfish—lobster, clams, shrimp, scallops, mussels, oysters, steamed, fried, in a sauce

Chicken—fried, broiled, baked, roasted, grilled

Beef—loin, strips, shanks, steaks, grilled, ground, roasted

Veal—grilled, roasted, marinated, breaded

Lamb—grilled, roasted, marinated

Sausage—grilled, sautéed

Pork—grilled, roasted, pulled, marinated

Turkey—roasted, ground

Duck and game—roasted, sautéed

Rice—fried, steamed

Potatoes—boiled, mashed, baked, french-fried, roasted, knishes, with gravy

Corn—steamed, steamed with butter, creamed, on the cob

Vegetables—artichokes, asparagus, avocados, broccoli, cabbage, carrots, cauliflower, celery, cucumbers, eggplant, fresh herbs, leafy greens, green beans, lettuce, mushrooms, onions and garlic, peppers, root vegetables (parsnips, beets, etc.), sprouts, squash, tomatoes, zucchini

Fast food

Burgers

Fries

Shakes

Cheap Mexican

Chinese

Movie nachos

Egg rolls

Lo mein

Quesadillas

McDonald's and Burger King burgers and fries

Processed cheese snacks—anything and everything that comes wrapped in paper, Styrofoam, or plastic and has lots of fat and chemicals

The Inventory, Part III: Beginning to Draw the Picture

Take a piece of paper and make three columns, like this:

Gotta Have It (G)   Borderline (B)   Indifferent (I)

Now, referring to your inventory, Part I and Part II, go through this list and tally up each of these categories. How many "gotta have it" foods do you have? How many "borderline" and "indifferent"? Any surprises?

Next, go through the "gotta have it" and "borderline" lists and make a third list, grouping everything into the following categories. Again, be specific and write down the brand or kind you love:

Categories

1. Sugary carbohydrates: Cake, cookies, donuts, pastries, sugary cereals

2. Chocolate: Bars, sauce, milk, dark, milk

3. Candy: From gumdrops to butterscotch

4. Frozen desserts: Ice cream, frozen yogurt, ice cream sandwiches, popsicles

5. Sugar-laden drinks: Regular soda, fruit drinks, juices

6. Salty, crunchy snacks: Chips, pretzels, crackers

7. Savory carbohydrates: Pasta, rice, bread, pizza

8. Potato: French fries, baked, etc.

9. Fried foods

10. Cheese: Mozzarella, Cheddar, American, etc.

11. Nuts: This includes roasted, raw, and peanut butter

12. Fast food: This includes all varieties of take-out, drive-throughs

13. Any particular meal that has a grip on you: Macaroni and cheese, French toast, a particular sandwich

14. Anything else?

The Inventory, Part IV: How is it done?

The next step is to identify and record how you are eating the foods you just listed. One of the keys to your recovery is identifying the links between food and location that have been solidified by behavior. You have your Life Log. Go through the recorded days and see if you can identify how you eat. A few examples:

√ • Refrigerator eating: standing and eating ice cream in front of the refrigerator

√ • Cupboard or sink eating: standing by the kitchen sink, spooning things such as peanut butter, ice cream, jelly, cream cheese, ricotta cheese, Cool Whip, chocolate syrup, honey, or mayonnaise into your mouth or standing in front of your cupboard and eating handfuls of cereal, nuts, or crackers

• TV eating: eating chip after chip, pretzel after pretzel, cookie after cookie while being mesmerized by a TV show or sports

• Bed eating: cozy under a comforter, eating a bag of popcorn, pretzels, or a bowl of ice cream

• Car eating: snacking or sneaking food on your way home, on your way to the office, or as you cruise around town running errands

• Supply room eating: scarfing down a bag of M&Ms by the copy machine

√ • Desk eating: eating while you work (in fact, a desk drawer or two might be devoted to this habit)

- I-just-have-to-get-something-in-the-kitchen eating: while your family is eating or after dinner, running into the kitchen for an extra bite or a bite of something you really want to be eating

- Cleanup eating: picking, grazing while cleaning up after a meal

- Movie eating: you buy the big popcorn, candy, and a soda and eat like a metronome as you watch a movie

- Grocery shopping eating: you pull a bag of chips down, open it, and eat the entire bag while shopping

- Closet eating: hiding food in a closet, the attic, your bureau, under the couch, or in your purse and sneaking it while others are not around or not looking

How you eat your "gotta have it" and borderline foods is your fourth list.

The Inventory, Part V:
Drawing Your Current Food Blueprint

Now, I want you to go back through the third list one more time and write down next to each of the food groups how much you are eating. An entire bag? A box? Two plates' worth? Again, please know that I am not going to make you calculate calories or use these amounts to shame you or make you feel worse about your eating habits. This is merely the final shading needed for drawing a clear picture of your food blueprint.

By this time, you should be able to fill in the blanks in the following summary (members of the Clean Your Plate Club, you might want to add "and have trouble controlling portion sizes" when describing how you eat):

I wake up at _____ [time] craving _____ [food].

I eat _____ for breakfast.

Then I _____.
[Examples here might include "drive or take the bus to work,"
"do household chores," "spend my morning doing _____"]

Then _____ ["after breakfast," "at/around 11 A.M.," etc.] I crave _____ [food] and eat it in the _____ [location].

Then I eat _____ for lunch at the _____ [location].

Then I crave _____ [type of food: salty, crunchy, sweet, etc.] at _____ [time] and eat it in the _____ [location]. [Bingers, you may want to add the amount here.]

Then I crave _____ [food] before dinner and eat it in the _____ [location].

While cooking/before dinner, I snack on_____ [food].

Then I eat _____ [food] for dinner in _____ [location].

Then I crave _____ [food] after dinner and eat it while I _____ [activity and location]. [TV watchers, you may want to add a section on commercial breaks that goes like this: "During commercials and between shows, I run to the kitchen for more _____."]

Then I crave _____ [food] before bed.

I often go to sleep thinking about _____ [food, what you might eat the next day, feeling guilty].

Maybe I get up and eat _____ [food] in the middle of the night standing in front of or by the _____ [location].

Once you feel you have thoroughly and honestly completed the final phase of the inventory, congratulate yourself. You just did something only a small fraction of people do. Really looking at what you eat and how much and writing it down, which makes it all very real, is perhaps the hardest part of the entire process. But the good news is, you now have the blueprint that you will soon work to modify. Soon your blueprint will sound more like this:

I wake up feeling rested and healthy.

For breakfast, generally, I pour myself a cup of coffee and have either a protein shake or some lean protein and low-carb fruit to fuel my mind and body.

Midmorning, if I'm feeling an energy low, I will drink some water and have a healthy snack of a handful of nuts or raisins. Maybe I'll have a cup of tea.

At lunch, I eat a salad with lean protein and low-fat dressing. I will feel full and satisfied.

Midafternoon, I will have a small, healthy snack of carrots or a piece of fruit to fuel my body. If I'm feeling stressed, I may do a five-minute mini meditation just to center myself and remember that my health and well-being are more important than the deadline. (This meditation is the same one that you learned to do in this chapter.)

In the evening, I will walk for twenty minutes. It's not my favorite thing to do, but it makes me feel good. And it is nice to spend some time outside after being inside all day.

For dinner, I will have some lean protein, vegetables, and maybe some steamed rice.

If I go out with friends, I will not feel compelled to eat everything the restaurant serves me. I may take a doggie bag home, or not. Again, I will feel full and satisfied.

Instead of watching the tube, I will read or do something I used to love to do, or maybe just putz around the house and then head to bed.

Don't believe me? Read on.

Annie's Story

A year ago, Annie, a beautiful nineteen-year-old woman, walked into my office devastated by her freshman year of college. Instead of gaining the usual "freshman 15," she had put on 40 pounds.

An active athlete in high school, Annie had never had trouble with her weight. She had always been able to eat what she wanted, so this intense weight gain was a terrifying shock. She thought there was something truly wrong with her—her thyroid, diabetes, maybe even cancer. She called her mother and they went to see several doctors. Each doctor told Annie that she was obese and should just work on losing that weight. One doctor went so far as to say, "A girl your age shouldn't be dealing with this kind of weight." These words devastated Annie. She was humiliated and terrified. Fortunately, Annie's mother had a friend who was also a client of mine, so she got my number and told Annie to call.

When Annie came in, we talked about what, after years of health and no weight struggle, could cause this kind of sudden gain. After talking some more, Annie and I identified her two key problems. One, for the first time in her life, Annie was not playing on a team. After years of exercising two to three hours a day for a sport, Annie wasn't doing any physical activity! Unfortunately, while Annie's body had stopped, her brain had not. It was programmed to eat for an athlete and was continuing to tell her to eat oatmeal, three eggs, and two slices of toast at breakfast. In the past, this kind of calorie loading would be fine, as Annie would be burning it off. But without running around for three hours, it had no place to go but to her hips.

The second problem was the obvious stress of a new school and college life. But what was interesting about this was that Annie had found just one food to use as her stress reliever: peanut butter. While she had eaten peanut butter her entire life, Annie said that she felt as if she had discovered peanut butter for the first time in college. Apparently, her school's refectory had a bread bar that featured peanut butter, jelly, and Marshmallow Fluff, and Annie had developed a serious affection for peanut butter on bread. This was in addition to whatever entree was being served. Annie told me that she included at least three slices of bread with peanut butter at most meals. Considering the fact that just 2 tablespoons of peanut butter is 188 calories with 15.9 grams of fat and 150 milligrams of sodium, I calculated that Annie was consuming about 2,400 extra calories a day in peanut butter and bread alone!

She also told me that by the spring semester, she had a jar of peanut butter in her room "just in case" and that this need to have a jar around at all times scared her. She had never emotionally depended on food before. She told me that when she was around peanut butter, she felt helpless and out of control.

I explained that we all have different responses to the stress that change can bring and that without the emotional and physical release of exercise, her body had told her to use food. Then we talked about her new food blueprint. She asked me to make her feel averse to peanut butter. I told her that if we did this, peanut butter might make her gag or feel sick from now on. She said, "I don't care. I will do anything to stop this weight gain." I also suggested making bread have less of a draw. Annie was concerned because she didn't want to stop enjoying bread entirely, but I explained to her that reframing foods does not change the taste. It just reduces the magnetic pull. Once she understood this, she heartily agreed to limit bread. We also talked about her getting back into sports, as stopping something that had been a huge source of joy for her in high school was obviously a big loss for her emotionally and physically.

Annie saw me for two sessions. Through having a new blueprint and exercising again, she lost the 40 pounds and continues to take action to improve her health and well-being. But more importantly, she feels in control and at ease with peanut butter, bread, and herself.

Annie's story is further proof that everyone, including you, can do this. You can take the next big step, which is putting the work of Chapter 7 into action—writing the script, writing your new food blueprint, writing your future. Are you ready? Turn the page. . . .

Script I:
Drawing a
New Blueprint

Chapter Eight

The food that enters the mind must be watched
as closely as the food that enters the body.

—Pat Buchanan

You have done a ton of work in the last few chapters, looking at the history and current reality of your relationship with food. The good news is that this next chapter is fun. You get to dream, fantasize, imagine, and define your new relationship with food.

In my office, when I ask my clients to define their dream relationship with food, they become animated and excited. They, probably like you, have been dreaming about a different kind of relationship with food for a long time—imagining being able to easily resist ordering a side of french fries or mashed potatoes at a diner, or just taking a few fries and being satisfied; dreaming of the day when they did not feel gripped or pulled by chocolate, or could wake up and *want* to exercise; picturing themselves walking down the street wearing clothes in shapes and sizes they could only dream of wearing, their hair looking a certain way, feeling confident, at ease, happy with themselves and with the world. But the best part is that this no longer has to be a fantasy. As

120

you know, 96 percent of my clients do realize a new relationship with food, their health, and well-being.

From here on out, the work that needs to be done is much less self-reflective and more task-oriented. First, we will identify a new life and food blueprint that will encourage your brain to have a pattern that includes exercise or moving more as well as eating more lean protein, fruits, vegetables, and whole grains and drinking enough water. With that in mind, let's get to the first task.

Describing Your New Life

In Chapter 7, I gave you a long list of foods to inspire you to think of any and all foods that you have difficulty with. In this chapter, the list of foods is brief. The reason we keep this list general and unspecific is that we want to promote and reprogram your brain with the general parameters for healthy eating. I want you to gravitate toward a direction rather than a specific food. Part of a healthy diet is variety, and I always want my clients to be open to new foods. Moreover, it has been my experience that restrictions and specifications generally lead to feelings of deprivation and obsession, which would put you right back into another food struggle—the last thing any of us wants.

So go through this next list and identify the healthy foods that you like and can see yourself eating. The reason I say this is that, while powerful, medical hypnosis is not magical. For instance, if you cannot stand fish, including fish in your new food blueprint is not a good plan. Even if you think you should be eating fish, if your palate fundamentally rejects the taste or texture of fish, it will continue to reject it even after medical hypnosis. The reason for this is that *hypnosis can't make you do something if you truly don't want to do it*. Remember, the idea that hypnosis can be used as a tool to control comes from the stereotype of entertainment hypnosis. But if you are open to eating something like fish and feel that with just a little push you could eat it and enjoy it more, then by all means include it in your list and see if the Alpha Solution helps push you in that healthy direction.

As with the Inventory in Chapter 7, feel free to add to this list, including other low-fat foods that you like or feel you'll be inclined to eat. I want you to lose weight, not your taste buds. For instance, I'm not a huge fan of diet soda or sugar substitutes, but if you feel passionate about them, you can include them. As for adding things such as diet foods or low-fat diet cookies, I think you should try to make your list without them, as you will find that with the Alpha Solution, you will not miss or need substitutes. You will be full and satisfied without them.

Go ahead and put a check next to the foods you would like to be drawn to. I recommend that everyone check the first two items, especially water. These will be your foundation foods—your diet essentials—for your New Pantry and new life.

New Pantry

Water—mineral water, tap water, soda water

Tea—herbal, green, with lemon, etc.

Coffee—black or with low-fat milk

Low-fat condiments

Mustard

Salad dressing—vinaigrette, low-fat

Fresh salsa

Dairy

Milk—2%, 1%, nonfat

Cottage cheese—low-fat, fat-free

Yogurt—low-fat, fat-free

Whole grains

Oatmeal

Brown rice

Whole-grain or multigrain breads

Whole-grain salads such as tabouli

Lean protein

Egg whites, poached eggs, soft-boiled eggs

Veggie burgers (no bun)

Fish—broiled, steamed, poached, grilled

Chicken—broiled, baked, roasted, grilled

Lean beef—loin, strips, shanks, steaks, ground, grilled, roasted, broiled

Lamb—grilled, roasted

Pork

Turkey

Beans

Fruit

I recommend these fruits because they are lower in sugar and carbohydrates than other fruits. This said, if you can't stand these fruits or want to add others, please do.

Apples

Blueberries

Strawberries

Raspberries

Vegetables

Make a list of a few key vegetables that you feel you might eat. For example, leafy greens and asparagus are two options. And please know that while corn and potatoes are vegetables, they should not be named or encouraged, as they contain starch and are often troublesome trigger foods.

Artichokes

Asparagus

Avocados

Broccoli

Cabbage

Carrots

Cauliflower

Celery

Cucumbers

Eggplant

Fresh herbs

Leafy greens

Green beans

Mushrooms

Onions and garlic

Peppers

Root vegetables (parsnips, beets, etc.)

Sprouts

Squash

Tomatoes

Zucchini

Do you feel you have a good idea of your future pantry? Are you happy with it? If not, go back through and think about what you'd like to add or subtract. Once you are happy, hold on to this list of healthy foods. You will need it in a moment, when you are filling out the script.

New Active Life

Now, let's identify a form of exercise or two that you can imagine yourself engaging in at least three and up to six times a week, activities such as:

- Aerobics

- Basketball

- Biking

- Elliptical trainer or a similar machine

- Rowing

- Running

- Swimming

- Tennis

- Walking

- Yoga

Don't select a sport you have had difficulty with in the past, as your brain already has a pattern for not enjoying that activity and it will be something else for you to fight against. For instance, for the most part, I have always hated exercise (even when I was lifting weights). So when I had to select an exercise, it was really about what I could stand to do, which was walk on a treadmill for forty-five minutes every day. And that's what I have been doing for more than twenty years. Exercise still is not my favorite thing, but I am healthier and feel better because of it. This said, many of my clients do find that hypnosis draws them to exercise, and some even come to love it.

I should also add that if you are horrified by the idea of including a physical activity in your script, you do not absolutely have to include one, but know that this may limit your ultimate success. Eating less and with control will certainly lead to weight loss, but exercise will greatly further that weight loss and promote a stronger sense of health and well-being.

Drafting the First Script

We're now ready to personalize the first medical hypnosis script you will use to introduce a new food blueprint for healthy eating and living to your brain. I am including the entire script so you can see it, become familiar with it, and understand how it works. I will give you as much of a "play-by-play" as I can, explaining the purpose of the language and how it works.

Overall, this first script is devoted to telling the subconscious mind that there is going to be a change and then describing what that change is going to be. For instance, if a client has a problem with five foods, chocolate, cheese, bread, pasta, and potatoes, then the client and I will write a script that tells the subconscious mind that these five foods are no longer going to be a problem. The problem is in the past. As we discussed in Chapter 3, the second script will reinforce this idea and support new healthy behaviors.

This first self-hypnosis script has several sections. There are sections you will personalize and other sections that are general and standard for everyone. **It is important to note that the sections of this script that are standard for everyone should not be changed.** The language is specifically designed to help you reprogram your brain. Any time you change the language in part of the standard script, you are risking weakening its strength and effectiveness. In this chapter, these standard sections will be in italics. The sections that are not in italics are sections that we will go through together and tailor to your needs. For example, if you want to feel indifferent to Dove Bars, in the "I am indifferent to _____" sentence of the script, you will simply write "Dove Bars" in the blank.

Going forward, my play-by-play notes will be in bold. They are not part of the script, nor will they be included in your recording. They are simply here to give you a deeper understanding of the process.

Once we have personalized the script, you will be ready to put all your medical hypnosis knowledge and work into action.

Feel free to write directly in the book. If you don't, then photocopy this script and write on the copy. And know that this is a draft. You will have a chance to create an official Script I for recording in Chapter 9.

Personalizing the script

Part I

As you know by now, in medical hypnosis we capitalize on the brain's natural alpha state to reframe the challenging issues and introduce new healthy behaviors to the subconscious mind. As with the release, we will use the induction method to bring about the relaxed alpha state. As you experienced with the release, this induction is here to help guide you and your body to be relaxed and at ease. Keep in mind as you go through the script that anything in brackets is an action to be done, not read. For instance, when you see "[Pause]," pause for a moment while reading. For now, don't worry about how fast you need to read this or how you are going to record and listen to this. This version, with my play-by-play, is simply here for you to read, familiarize yourself with, and personalize.

The Induction

[Read]

Be sure you're in a comfortable position.

With your eyes closed.

The head and neck supported well.

Ready for sleep.

Remember, do not hesitate or prevent yourself from falling asleep while listening. Remember, the early stage of sleep is the deepest form of the alpha or hypnotic state. So I encourage you to fall asleep while listening.

[Pause]

Place one hand on your lower belly.

The reason for doing this is to be sure that you are breathing from your belly. Not your chest. Not your shoulders. Just the lower abdomen. Feel the belly rising and falling as you breathe. Your chest and shoulders should be relaxed and at ease.

Breathing in this way always helps induce relaxation and sleep.

Take a deep cleansing breath in through your nostrils.

And then a nice slow exhale through your mouth.

Just notice your hand rising and falling with each breath, indicating your belly is doing the work.

Take another deep cleansing breath in through your nostrils.

And a nice slow exhale through your mouth.

And repeat that one more time.

Inhale.

Exhale.

And when you complete this deep breath, continue to breathe in a normal fashion.

Through your nostrils.

If you have trouble breathing through your nostrils, then just breathe through your mouth.

And just continue to breathe normally.

Observe the flow of air coming in and out, while focused on the sound of your voice.

Try to leave the rest of the world on hold. And just be focused on your own words.

[Pause]

To help relax further:

Tense up all the muscles in your forehead.

Squeeze your eyes shut so they're squinched up as tightly closed as possible.

Clench your teeth tightly.

Now tense up all the facial muscles.

Tighten them.

Hold that.

A little tighter.

Tighter.

Tighter.

And relax, letting your facial muscles go.

Breathe.

Inhale.

Exhale.

Good.

Notice how good the facial muscles feel, so relaxed.

Now, be sure your head is supported well. No strain on your neck or back.

Let your head just feel heavy, supported, tension-free, easy.

Now, raise your shoulders toward your ears as if you're trying to touch your earlobes.

Higher.

Higher.

Higher.

And let them drop, like they have weights pressing on them.

Nice and heavy and relaxed.

Let them go.

Inhale.

Exhale.

Good.

Now, I want you to think of yourself as being as relaxed as a rag doll.

In fact, use that image.

Imagine you're looking at a rag doll just slumped in a chair.

Totally effortless.

Completely relaxed.

Imagine being that comfortable and relaxed.

Hold that image and thought in your mind as you continue to relax further.

Now tense up all the muscles in your arms.

Make fists.

Squeeze.

Tighter.

Tighter.

Tighter.

And release.

Relax.

Let those arms just drop and relax, like heavy weights.

Let them feel heavy.

Now bear down on the belly.

Tighten up on the abdominal muscles.

Squeezing.

Tighter.

Tighter.

Tighter.

And relax.

Take a deep breath in through your nose.

And a nice long exhale through your mouth.

Let go of any remaining tension.

Drift and relax.

And finally, tense up all the muscles in your legs, from the buttocks all the way to the toes.

Tense your thighs.

Point your toes. Straight out.

Tense your calves.

Hold that.

Tighter.

Tighter.

Tighter.

And let them drop.

Nice and heavy.

Like logs.

And relax.

Take another deep breath in through your nostrils.

And exhale, letting the breath out through your mouth, nice and slow.

Let it all go.

Notice how the body feels now.

How relaxed.

Like a rag doll.

Notice how slow your breathing has become and how much slower it will be over the next few minutes. Notice how cool the air is on your inhale and how warm it is when you exhale.

Good.

The body has moved into a meditative, profoundly relaxed state and will continue to do so with each breath.

This is known as the alpha state. This is when the subconscious mind is most open and most receptive to the information that comes in. In this case, your newly established relationship with food will be imprinted. You will no longer struggle with food.

Use your imagination now.

Picture everything that is now being described.

Imagine you're at the top of a staircase.

There are ten stairs going down below you.

Picture yourself at the top of the staircase.

See yourself the way you want to look.

Lean.

Strong.

Healthy.

Get a good picture of yourself.

Make sure you see your face as clearly as you can. Know that it is you who looks so great.

See the outline of your body exactly as you want it to be.

Lean.

Strong.

Healthy.

Get a vivid picture in your mind's eye.

This picture is not as a result of a diet or struggle or the feeling of being deprived.

In fact, it is the result of the opposite of feeling deprived.

This picture of you,

lean,

strong,

and healthy,

is a result of a new healthy relationship with food where you are in control.

And free of the struggle.

You feel empowered.

Picture yourself now,

lean,

strong,

and healthy,

at the top of the stairs with this feeling of empowerment and self-respect for your mind and body.

As you hear the counting from ten to one, picture yourself taking a corresponding step down those stairs.

[Read steadily]

Ten.

Nine.

Each step a little more relaxed than before.

Eight.

More focused.

Seven.

Deeper and deeper relaxation.

Six.

Five.

Four.

Three.

Two.

One.

Bottom of the stairs.

Anytime you hear yourself count from ten to one while picturing yourself going down those stairs, you'll enter a deeper, more focused alpha state and become more receptive than the time before.

[End of the induction]

This next section is called the Reframe. It is similar to the release you did in Chapter 5. In the Release, you used language and imagery to let go of your history with food, including the messages about food and eating you heard as a child. In the reframe, we use language and imagery to tell your brain:

1. That there is going to be a change

2. To put food in its proper place and size

3. To let go and reject any and all current unhealthy behaviors and problem foods that challenge and taunt you

4. **That the struggle with food is in the past and that you are now in total control of the food you put in your body**

5. **That there is a new, healthy food picture**

The Reframe

I want you to imagine now that you're in a very large field.

The sky is blue. Not a cloud in sight.

The grass is an emerald green.

It's soft under your feet.

This big field is surrounded by beautiful, tall trees.

The trees are swaying in a warm, delicious breeze.

You are the only person there.

Across the field in the center you see a hot-air balloon.

Give the balloon a color.

Picture yourself walking toward the balloon.

See it more clearly now.

Soon you are close enough to make out the texture on the balloon's wicker basket.

Fill in all the details of what the basket looks like.

See that the balloon is full and ready to go.

Notice that the only thing preventing the basket from floating away are four sandbags, one on the rim of each side of the wicker basket.

Now you are so close that you can look up into the balloon and see inside it.

Now look inside the basket.

Other than the propane tank that fuels the hot air, it is empty.

The basket is ready for its load.

Now I want you to put all of your unhealthy behaviors in the basket.

This language reinforces the Release, reminding the brain that you have released all the behaviors you identified in Chapter 5 and let go in Chapter 6. See yourself putting these behaviors—cravings for crap, cleaning your plate, eating as soon as you walk in the door, believing food is love, stress eating, and so on—into the basket. Use as many of the "See yourself" phrases as you need to create a complete script that directly addresses all your food issues and behaviors. I've included ten to get you started. And please, if you need to jog your memory by referring back to Chapters 5 and 6, please do so.

See yourself putting _____ in the basket.

See yourself putting _____ in the basket.

See yourself putting _____ in the basket.

See yourself putting _____ in the basket.

See yourself putting _____ in the basket.

See yourself putting _____ in the basket.

See yourself putting _____ in the basket.

See yourself putting _____ in the basket.

See yourself putting _____ in the basket.

See yourself putting _____ in the basket.

Now, I want you to picture yourself putting the foods you struggle with into the basket.

This is where the information from the third part of your Inventory in Chapter 7 belongs (p. 113). List the foods here. For instance, I included potatoes, pizza, and bread. Use as many of the "See yourself" phrases as you need to—I've included ten to get you started, but take all the space you need. The basket can hold as much as you need it to. Remember to be specific with what you are putting into the basket. For instance, if Sprite is one of your foods, don't say "soda," say "Sprite."

See yourself putting _____ in the basket.

See yourself putting _____ in the basket.

See yourself putting _____ in the basket.

See yourself putting _____ in the basket.

See yourself putting _____ in the basket.

See yourself putting _____ in the basket.

See yourself putting _____ in the basket.

See yourself putting _____ in the basket.

See yourself putting _____ in the basket.

See yourself putting _____ in the basket.

Notice that there is space for all these foods in the basket.

When you are done putting the food and unhealthy habits and behaviors in the basket, look into the basket and see that this basket holds your entire struggle with food.

The struggle is no longer part of you.

Your old relationship with food—the struggle—is in this basket.

The foods and behaviors have been compartmentalized.

They are separate from you.

Not part of you in any way.

Everything you need and want to be free of is now in the basket.

It is now in its rightful and proper place.

Now, I want you to notice a giant picnic blanket draped near one of the sandbags.

Give it a color.

Give it a texture.

Now, I want to see you pulling it down off the sides of the basket and draping it over the contents of the basket.

So that you can no longer see your struggle.

Notice that this blanket is heavy enough to not blow away.

It settles on top of the contents of the basket and stays there, sealing them in.

Making the separation between you and your struggle even more solid, permanent.

I want you to use your inner voice now.

Repeat each of the following phrases exactly like this.

Begin with the following:

Any overwhelming desire for overindulging exists sealed in the basket.

This language addresses overeating for members of the Clean Your Plate Club.

Any desire for food when there is no physiological need to eat exists sealed in the basket.

This language addresses snacking, craving, and binging.

This next section, which is part of the script's Reframe, is where you will include the foods you identified in the third part of your Inventory in Chapter 7 (p. 113). Note: If you do not have an issue with salty, crunchy foods for example, you can cross this sentence out. Fill in:

Any overwhelming desire for _____ [Write in all the sugary carbohydrates—cakes, cookies, donuts, pastries, sugary cereals— that challenge you] exists sealed in the basket.

Any overwhelming desired for _____ [Write in all forms of chocolate that challenge you] exists sealed in the basket.

Any overwhelming desire for _____ [Write in all kinds of candy that challenge you] exists sealed in the basket.

Any overwhelming desire for _____ [Write in all frozen desserts that challenge you—ice cream and frozen yogurt] exists sealed in the basket.

Any overwhelming desire for _____ [Write in all sodas and sugar-laden drinks, including juice, that challenge you] exists sealed in the basket.

Any overwhelming desire for _____ [Write in all the salty, crunchy snacks that challenge you] exists sealed in the basket.

Any overwhelming desire for _____ [Write in all the kinds of savory carbohydrates—rice, pasta, bread, and pizza—that challenge you] exists sealed in the basket.

Any overwhelming desire for _____ [Write in your list of all the variations of potato that challenge you] exists sealed in the basket.

Any overwhelming desire for _____ [Write in your list of favorite fried foods] exists sealed in the basket.

Any overwhelming desire for _____ [Write in all the cheeses that challenge you] exists sealed in the basket.

Any overwhelming desire for _____ [Write in all varieties and variations of nuts that challenge you—nuts to peanut and almond butter] exists sealed in the basket.

Any overwhelming desire for _____ [Write in all varieties and brands of fast food that challenge you] exists sealed in the basket.

Any overwhelming desire for _____ [Write in all varieties and kinds of meals that challenge you] exists sealed in the basket.

Now, the standard script continues.

Any use of food in a hurtful way exists sealed in the basket.

This language addresses those messages such as deprivation, food is love, eating to please, eating as revenge or armor or to relieve stress (as you now know, it only adds to stress and thus is hurtful).

Everything in the basket is in its rightful place.

I cannot miss what I no longer want.

My conscious, logical desires are represented in the basket, so my conscious and subconscious desires are in sync—there is no more ambivalence.

I am in total control of my relationship with food.

[End use of inner voice. Read on.]

So the conscious and subconscious minds are synchronized now. They both want you to be

lean,

strong,

and healthy.

Without feeling deprived, without dieting—in fact, feeling empowered.

Now, I want you to imagine yourself standing next to that basket.

So that you're right there in front of it.

So that the giant balloon is truly looming over you.

You're seeing it.

You're looking up at it.

It's towering over you.

Know that the basket and the balloon hold everything that blocks you from realizing your potential.

Look up and see the field.

See the wide-open potential that lies before you.

Now bring your attention back to the basket.

See the four sandbags.

One draped over each of the four sides of the basket.

They are the only things holding this basket and all your struggles in place.

See that you have the power and strength to move them.

To push them to the ground.

To release your struggle.

The release of this basket is the end of the struggle.

Your freedom, health, and well-being are waiting for you.

Now imagine yourself pushing the first sandbag off the edge of the basket.

See the basket and balloon shift.

Move to another side of the basket and push another sandbag off.

The basket is now pulling up, almost free.

Move to another sandbag. Push the third bag off.

The basket is lifting off.

Run to the final side of the basket.

Release the sandbag.

See the balloon lift off.

Float up.

Carrying away the struggle with it.

It is above the trees now.

It is getting higher and higher.

Floating away beyond the edge of the field.

Watch it go.

See it getting smaller and smaller.

It is now only a speck on the horizon.

And then,

it is gone.

You can no longer see it.

How can something you can no longer see have any control over you?

It can't.

The basket with all that it contains is completely powerless over you.

It is gone.

You cannot see it.

The struggle is in its proper place. There is no ambivalence about this. It has been eradicated from your life.

You have reframed your relationship to food.

You have taken control of your life.

Now, see yourself taking your experience to the next logical level.

Picture yourself

lean,

strong,

and healthy.

Free of the balloon and all that it represents.

Feel and see how good that feels.

You have that entire field to yourself.

Jump around.

Dance.

Sing.

Feel the freedom from the burden.

Feel empowered. Feel in control of food.

You have not only contained the struggle, you have let it go.

And as you continue to enjoy your freedom, repeat this phrase in your inner voice: "_____." [Write your Anchor Statement you used in your Release here. For example, "I control food. Food does not control me."]

Now that you're past your struggle, know that the balloon and all your food issues are behind you.

Every time you reexperience this metaphor of a balloon floating away, the subconscious mind knows exactly what it means.

The struggle is over. You're more free of it with every repetition of the balloon floating away.

The phrase "_____" [Use your Anchor Statement here.] will forever be linked to the freedom, the fact that you can walk past any old nemesis with ease.

The struggle is gone. It has floated away.

Anytime you use the phrase "_____" [Use your Anchor Statement here.] you are reminding the subconscious mind that you are in control of what, when, where, why, and how much you eat.

Reminder: Your Anchor Statement is the key, the linchpin to your success. Do not change this phrase when recording the script or when saying it to yourself, ever. After listening to the script, when you say this phrase to yourself, it will connect you to the script, the experience, and your new subconscious desire to be lean, strong, and healthy. It is the link to your new food blueprint. You can say it to yourself if you have a craving, standing in line, at the theater, at the office, and always before you eat.

So the phrase and the metaphor of freeing the balloon are one and the same.

The phrase becomes a conditioned response.

Each time you use the phrase, it will trigger an automatic reflex, the instinct to make a healthy choice for mind and body.

This picture of the balloon floating away matches your conscious desire to be free of the struggle and be

lean,

strong,

and healthy.

Your conscious and subconscious minds are in agreement.

You are free of ambivalence.

Your conscious desire to be

lean,

strong,

and healthy

is reflected by your subconscious response to produce this healthy desire.

Every time you use the phrase "_____" [Use your Anchor Statement here.] you want to make the healthy choice for mind and body.

To become and remain lean, strong, and healthy.

Repeat each of the following phrases in your inner voice:

"_____" [Use your Anchor Statement here.] I feel full and satisfied with moderate portions at meals.

Again, this language reinforces eating in moderation for those who overeat and are members of the Clean Your Plate Club.

Food is fuel for health and well-being.

This language reinforces the idea that you need to eat only when you are hungry.

If there's no need to refuel, then there's no desire for eating.

This language reinforces the idea that snacking, stress eating, or eating for any purpose other than satisfying hunger is not necessary.

I refuel only when there's a physiological need.

This next section refers to the same Inventory from Chapter 7 that you've already used once. Note that the language is a bit different. The struggle is now in the past. You have reframed the struggle.

I am completely indifferent to _____. [Write in all the sugary carbohydrates—cakes, cookies, donuts, pastries, and sugary cereals—that challenged you.] I can bypass this/them anytime.

I am completely indifferent to _____. [Write in all forms of chocolate that challenged you.] I can bypass this/them anytime.

I am completely indifferent to _____. [Write in all kinds of candy that challenged you.] I can bypass this/them anytime.

I am completely indifferent to _____. [Write in all frozen desserts that challenged you—ice cream and frozen yogurt.] I can bypass this/them anytime.

I am completely indifferent to _____. [Write in all sodas and sugar-laden drinks, including juice, that challenged you.] I can bypass this/them anytime.

I am completely indifferent to _____. [Write in all the salty, crunchy snacks that challenged you.] I can bypass this/them anytime.

I am completely indifferent to _____. [Write in all the kinds of savory carbohydrates—pasta, pizza, and bread—that challenged you.] I can bypass this/them anytime.

I am completely indifferent to _____. [Write in your list of all the variations of potato that challenged you.] I can bypass this/them anytime.

I am completely indifferent to _____. [Write in your list of favorite fried foods that challenged you.] I can bypass this/them anytime.

I am completely indifferent to _____. [Write in all the cheeses that challenged you.] I can bypass this/them anytime.

I am completely indifferent to _____. [Write in all varieties and variations of nuts that challenged you—nuts to peanut and almond butter.] I can bypass this/them anytime.

I am completely indifferent to _____. [Write in all varieties and brands of fast food that challenged you.] I can bypass this/them anytime.

I am completely indifferent to _____. [Write in all varieties and kinds of meals that challenged you.] I can bypass this/them anytime.

I reject using food in a hurtful way.

Again, this reinforces the idea that we eat for our health and well-being. Not to get back at our parents or siblings, not for any other reason.

Because I care for my mind and body as I would care for any precious life.

I am a precious life and I use food accordingly.

I would no sooner use food to hurt myself than use it to hurt any innocent life.

I cannot miss what I no longer desire.

I am empowered over food. Never deprived of it.

The only substitute I need is the phrase "_____." [Use your Anchor Statement here.]

The phrase and my healthy relationship with food are one and the same.

The phrase represents the healthy, empowering use of food.

The phrase becomes more effective every day, with every use of it.

The phrase helps me feel comfortable from within, positive, and energized.

The phrase helps me become and remain lean, strong, and healthy.

[Note: End of using the inner voice. The following text is a narrative for you to read and then listen to.]

Now, picture yourself free of the struggle.

Feel the strength you have.

Feel how good it feels to have eliminated the struggle, to be on a supportive path of health and well-being.

You're on your way to becoming and remaining

lean,

strong,

and healthy.

Picture yourself in the field looking

lean,

strong,

and healthy.

Feeling unencumbered. Unblocked.

Each time you experience this you put the struggle further and further behind you.

You are closer to being healthy, happy, joyous, and free.

The New Blueprint

This next section is devoted to showing your brain a new blueprint—a new picture and idea of life and your future. This is the dress rehearsal for your future reality. Every time you rehearse this picture, the more natural the inclination will be to realize it in life. The line between fantasy and life will dwindle away. The more you reexperience it in your imagination, the more it becomes a part of you. If you reproduce this picture every day, you will soon wake up wanting to do it. You will live it.

Now I want you to picture yourself walking to the end of the field.

When you arrive, see a path.

Now really see that path.

This is the path to health and well-being.

Let the path stand out.

Give it a color.

Give it a texture.

Picture it raised so that it is slightly above the level of the ground you are standing on.

The path is still secure, but it is on a higher plane.

Step up onto this path.

This is the path that leads to your health and well-being.

It is never-ending.

Start walking.

Give the path a scent.

Inhale the sweetness.

Picture yourself being on a higher plane.

Caring for yourself.

See yourself going through your day choosing the healthy foods you have identified.

[Include a few key foods from your New Pantry in the first blanks and two key trouble foods from your inventory in Chapter 7 in the second blank. For example, "Choosing salad instead of grilled cheese."]

Choosing _____ *instead of* _____.

Choosing _____ *instead of* _____.

Eating _____. [Insert a healthy food from your New Pantry list in this chapter.]

Drinking water.

Picture yourself _____. [Insert exercise activity you chose earlier in this chapter—for example, walking, swimming, biking.]

You are doing this for your mind. Your body.

You are on a higher level.

The path is forever associated with the phrase
"_____." [Use your Anchor Statement here.] *Regardless of the path others choose, you crave the path that's right for you.*

The color you have given your path is also forever linked to this phrase. So every time you see the color, it will reinforce your new relationship with food.

The path and the phrase are one and the same.

Now picture yourself walking on that path.

Picture yourself moving forward at a healthy pace.

You're lighter.

You're not carrying the weight.

The weight is off you.

The struggle is off you.

You took control of it.

It is gone.

There is nothing blocking you or weighing you down.

You are unblocked, unencumbered.

The field is further and further behind you.

Like anything else, the further you walk away from something, the smaller it gets.

In fact, you have walked so far along this path of health and well-being that you cannot even see the field.

The field is out of sight.

And so is the balloon.

If you were to glance back to look for it, you couldn't even see it with binoculars.

It is gone.

You are making your way on the path of empowerment. Of health and well-being.

The path is always with you and always supporting you.

The path of health and well-being is endless.

Picture it going into the horizon.

Never-ending.

The path is representative of your foundation foods.

The foods that you crave in moderate portions. The path where food is fuel for health, enjoyment, and self-respect.

This next section lists your new foods that you would like to encourage your brain to be inclined to crave and eat. Refer to the New Pantry list from this chapter and specify which lean proteins, fruits, vegetables, salads, whole grains, and healthy condiments you would like to be eating more of. Fill in the blanks as you go.

Lean proteins such as _____. This is/they are represented by the path.

Fruits such as _____. This is/they are represented by the path.

Vegetables such as _____. This is/they are represented by the path.

Whole grains such as _____. This is/they are represented by the path.

Condiments such as _____. This is/they are represented by the path.

Dairy products such as _____. This is/they are represented by the path.

Beverages such as _____. This is/they are represented by the path.

Water.

And other healthy choices that fuel your mind and body in an appropriate way.

Every breath you draw,

every step you take,

brings you closer to optimal health and joy.

Lean,

strong,

and healthy.

As you progress forward, think of all the positive things that come with being on the path of health and well-being.

Self-respect.

Ease.

Contentment.

Joy.

Freedom.

Your loved ones.

Health.

Well-being.

*Feeling good, every day, all day, from within, **not** from an external source such as food.*

Continue to picture these things.

Stay with this picture.

Stay with these feelings of love, ease, and contentment until you fall into a very

[Read slowly]

deep,

sound sleep.

[End of script]

_____

So, how did it go? Pretty simple, right? Now it's time to take the next step. If you feel you have included all the foods you want to reframe and have a good idea of the foods and life you want to live with in the future, you are now ready to record your script. Let's move on!

Recording
Script I

Chapter Nine

He is not happy who does not realize his happiness.

—Latin proverb

Now it's time to make all your work real. In this chapter, we're going to put your vision for your future self on record—on a CD or MP3.

In my sessions, I read and record the same basic script we devised in Chapter 8 for my clients. But in this book I am asking you to read and record your own script, and doing it is very important. For one thing, as we've seen, it's crucial that your script be customized to treat *you* and your specific food issues and behaviors. You can find dozens of generic audio hypnosis weight-loss CDs on the Web and in stores. In my experience, these generic recordings are largely useless. As you learned in Chapter 4, general language doesn't treat specific food problems. The subconscious mind is literal. Chocolate is chocolate, not candy.

The second reason why it is critical to do it on your own is so that your subconscious mind responds as fully and deeply as possible. In my sessions, I ask my clients to use their inner voice and repeat statements after me because I know their subconscious minds might reject a state-ment such as "I control food. Food cannot control me" in my unfamiliar voice. The subconscious mind will tune in and be more willing to accept the new blueprint when it is delivered in a familiar voice the subconscious mind can trust. So by having you reading the suggestions with your own voice and then repeating them using your inner voice, you are telling your subconscious mind to change twice. And, as you have learned, the more the subconscious mind hears an idea, the more it will make that idea reality. So while recording your own script is more work, the use of your voice in a self-hypnosis recording makes the treat-ment that much more powerful and effective.

How to Record the First Script

Creating your personalized medical hypnosis script does not require a recording studio, a producer, or even much effort. It's as simple as slowly reading the script into any kind of recording device. In today's world, the recording options are endless. Most are inexpensive and all are very easy. A few suggestions:

- Record the script into a microcassette recorder.

- Record the script using a regular cassette recorder.

- Record the script onto CD using your stereo and a microphone.

- Record the script on your computer and then burn a CD or transfer the recording to your iPod. There are hundreds of Web sites devoted to telling you how you can use your home com-puter technology to record. A couple of good Web sites include http://www.ehow.com/how_10021_record-sound-windows.htm and www.wikihow.com/Record-a-CD.

- Use a digital audiotape (DAT) recorder.

Please do not invest in some new expensive machine whose abilities and strengths you can barely comprehend, or struggle to master an overwhelmingly complex sound technology. When choosing the medium you are going to use, be sure to select a level of technology and machine that you feel comfortable with. That said, I do want you to strive for the best recording possible. This means that you should:

Give yourself at least an hour to record the script.

The actual reading of the script should take roughly twenty minutes, but I suggest recording yourself a few times as practice so that you can find your rhythm and identify the parts where you need to either speed up or slow down. Then, after half an hour or so of experimenting, you can make your "official" recording. Giving yourself this hour is giving yourself the road to freedom.

Record the script in a quiet place.

Because you want your subconscious mind to hear the message you have recorded and nothing else, the quieter the background, the better. Be sure to note that the more sensitive the technology you are using, the more extraneous noise it will catch. For instance, a DAT device will probably pick up the background noises that things such as refrigerators and fluorescent lights make. So be sure to be aware of what is around you—street noise, the children downstairs, a TV in the background, doors opening and closing, hum from lights, birds, dogs barking, and so on. One obvious and excellent way to ensure that you have the clean background you want is to listen to one of your test recordings and to see if you hear anything between your words. You may find that your closet (if it has a light and is big enough) is as good a place as any for quiet, solitude, and focus. Don't forget to turn off your phone's ringer!

Know that it does not have to be perfect.

Okay, I know that in Chapter 7 I said that you cannot change the script and must follow it to the letter or else it will hinder your ability to change your established blueprint. This is true—to a point. If, as you are recording the script, you find yourself changing a word here or there unconsciously or because you have a terrible association with a word or just don't like it, please change it. Or if you find yourself adding imagery to the balloon section of the script, by all means go ahead. **This said, you may not change the language in the script where you use your inner voice. Nor can you change the Anchor Statement you used in your Release.** As I've said, these phrases are the foundation of the script and of your recovery.

Other than these three guiding principles, there is really nothing more you need to know about recording your script. Overall, my main piece of advice for you is to have fun with it. Enjoy the process. Know that it is the key to the end of your struggle with food. Perhaps think of it as a ritual, or just as a giant step toward the rest of the big and beautiful life you have ahead of you. It's okay if you stumble over a word or say "um" here and there. Don't strive for perfection—just relax and read the script at a slow but steady pace.

I am including another copy of the script here. Again, you can write directly in the book or make a copy and write on that. It's up to you. This version does not have my play-by-play comments in it, so it will be easier for you to read and record. **Go through this version and add in your Anchor Statement and the personal details that you identi-fied in Chapters 7 and 8.** This is your final opportunity to review the work you've done. Take a moment to ask yourself, "Have I included everything? Are all the foods and behaviors listed?" If so, then you are ready to go on record with your new food blueprint.

Reminder: Anything in brackets is an action to be done, not read. For instance, when you see "[Pause]," pause for a moment while read-ing. **As you are reading, remember to relax and breathe! Sound like your natural self!**

The First Script

[Read at a slow and steady pace]

Be sure you're in a comfortable position.

With your eyes closed.

The head and neck supported well.

Ready for sleep.

Remember, do not hesitate or prevent yourself from falling asleep while listening. Remember, the early stage of sleep is the deepest form of the alpha or hypnotic state. So I encourage you to fall asleep while listening.

[Pause]

Place one hand on your lower belly.

The reason for doing this is to be sure that you are breathing from your belly. Not your chest. Not your shoulders. Just the lower abdomen. Feel the belly rising and falling as you breathe. Your chest and shoulders should be relaxed and at ease.

Breathing in this way always helps induce relaxation and sleep.

Take a deep cleansing breath in through your nostrils.

And then a nice slow exhale through your mouth.

Just notice your hand rising and falling with each breath, indicating your belly is doing the work.

Take another deep cleansing breath in through your nostrils.

And a nice slow exhale through your mouth.

And repeat that one more time.

Inhale.

Exhale.

And when you complete this deep breath, continue to breathe in a normal fashion.

Through your nostrils.

If you have trouble breathing through your nostrils, then just breathe through your mouth.

And just continue to breathe normally.

Observe the flow of air coming in and out, while focused on the sound of your voice.

Try to leave the rest of the world on hold. And just be focused on your own words.

[Pause]

To help relax further:

Tense up all the muscles in your forehead.

Squeeze your eyes shut so they're squinched up as tightly closed as possible.

Clench your teeth tightly.

Now tense up all the facial muscles.

Tighten them.

Hold that.

A little tighter.

Tighter.

Tighter.

And relax, letting your facial muscles go.

Breathe.

Inhale.

Exhale.

Good.

Notice how good the facial muscles feel, so relaxed.

Now, be sure your head is supported well. No strain on your neck or back.

Let your head just feel heavy, supported, tension-free, easy.

Now, raise your shoulders toward your ears as if you're trying to touch your earlobes.

Higher.

Higher.

Higher.

And let them drop, like they have weights pressing on them.

Nice and heavy and relaxed.

Let them go.

Inhale.

Exhale.

Good.

Now, I want you to think of yourself as being as relaxed as a rag doll.

In fact, use that image.

Imagine you're looking at a rag doll just slumped in a chair.

Totally effortless.

Completely relaxed.

Imagine being that comfortable and relaxed.

Hold that image and thought in your mind as you continue to relax further.

Now tense up all the muscles in your arms.

Make fists.

Squeeze.

Tighter.

Tighter.

Tighter.

And release.

Relax.

Let those arms just drop and relax, like heavy weights.

Let them feel heavy.

Now bear down on the belly.

Tighten up on the abdominal muscles.

Squeezing.

Tighter.

Tighter.

Tighter.

And relax.

Take a deep breath in through your nose.

And a nice long exhale through your mouth.

Let go of any remaining tension.

Drift and relax.

And finally, tense up all the muscles in your legs, from the buttocks all the way to the toes.

Tense your thighs.

Point your toes. Straight out.

Tense your calves.

Hold that.

Tighter.

Tighter.

Tighter.

And let them drop.

Nice and heavy.

Like logs.

And relax.

Take another deep breath in through your nostrils.

And exhale, letting the breath out through your mouth, nice and slow.

Let it all go.

Notice how the body feels now.

How relaxed.

Like a rag doll.

Notice how slow your breathing has become and how much slower it will be over the next few minutes. Notice how cool the air is on your inhale and how warm it is when you exhale.

Good.

The body has moved into a meditative, profoundly relaxed state and will continue to do so with each breath.

This is known as the alpha state. This is when the subconscious mind is most open and most receptive to the information that comes in. In this case, your newly established relationship with food will be imprinted. You will no longer struggle with food.

Use your imagination now.

Picture everything that is now being described.

Imagine you're at the top of a staircase.

There are ten stairs going down below you.

Picture yourself at the top of the staircase.

See yourself the way you want to look.

Lean.

Strong.

Healthy.

Get a good picture of yourself.

Make sure you see your face as clearly as you can. Know that it is you who looks so great.

See the outline of your body exactly as you want it to be.

Lean.

Strong.

Healthy.

Get a vivid picture in your mind's eye.

This picture is not as a result of a diet or struggle or the feeling of being deprived.

In fact, it is the result of the opposite of feeling deprived.

This picture of you,

lean,

strong,

and healthy,

is a result of a new healthy relationship with food where you are in control.

And free of the struggle.

You feel empowered.

Picture yourself now,

lean,

strong,

and healthy,

at the top of the stairs with this feeling of empowerment and self-respect for your mind and body.

As you hear the counting from ten to one, picture yourself taking a corresponding step down those stairs.

[Read steadily]

Ten.

Nine.

Each step a little more relaxed than before.

Eight.

More focused.

Seven.

Deeper and deeper relaxation.

Six.

Five.

Four.

Three.

Two.

One.

Bottom of the stairs.

Anytime you hear yourself count from ten to one while picturing yourself going down those stairs, you'll enter a deeper, more focused alpha state and become more receptive than the time before.

[End of Induction]

[Pause]

I want you to imagine now that you're in a very large field.

The sky is blue. Not a cloud in sight.

The grass is an emerald green.

It's soft under your feet.

This big field is surrounded by beautiful, tall trees.

The trees are swaying in a warm, delicious breeze.

You are the only person there.

Across the field in the center you see a hot-air balloon.

Give the balloon a color.

Picture yourself walking toward the balloon.

See it more clearly now.

Soon you are close enough to make out the texture on the balloon's wicker basket.

Fill in all the details of what the basket looks like.

See that the balloon is full and ready to go.

Notice that the only thing preventing the basket from floating away are four sandbags, one on the rim of each side of the wicker basket.

Now you are so close that you can look up into the balloon and see inside it.

Now look inside the basket.

Other than the propane tank that fuels the hot air, it is empty.

The basket is ready for its load.

Now I want you to put all of your unhealthy behaviors in the basket.

See yourself putting _____ in the basket.

See yourself putting _____ in the basket.

See yourself putting _____ in the basket.

See yourself putting _____ in the basket.

See yourself putting _____ in the basket.

See yourself putting _____ in the basket.

See yourself putting _____ in the basket.

See yourself putting _____ in the basket.

See yourself putting _____ in the basket.

See yourself putting _____ in the basket.

Now, I want you to picture yourself putting the foods you struggle with into the basket.

See yourself putting _____ in the basket.

See yourself putting _____ in the basket.

See yourself putting _____ in the basket.

See yourself putting _____ in the basket.

See yourself putting _____ in the basket.

See yourself putting _____ in the basket.

See yourself putting _____ in the basket.

See yourself putting _____ in the basket.

See yourself putting _____ in the basket.

Notice that there is space for all these foods in the basket.

When you are done putting the food and unhealthy habits and behaviors in the basket, look into the basket and see that this basket holds your entire struggle with food.

The struggle is no longer part of you.

Your old relationship with food—the struggle—is in this basket.

The foods and behaviors have been compartmentalized.

They are separate from you.

Not part of you in any way.

Everything you need and want to be free of is now in the basket.

It is now in its rightful and proper place.

Now, I want you to notice a giant picnic blanket draped near one of the sandbags.

Give it a color.

Give it a texture.

Now, I want to see you pulling it down off the sides of the basket and draping it over the contents of the basket.

So that you can no longer see your struggle.

Notice that this blanket is heavy enough to not blow away.

It settles on top of the contents of the basket and stays there, sealing them in.

Making the separation between you and your struggle even more solid, permanent.

I want you to use your inner voice now.

Repeat each of the following phrases exactly like this.

Begin with the following:

Any overwhelming desire for overindulging exists sealed in the basket.

Any desire for food when there is no medicinal need to eat exists sealed in the basket.

Any overwhelming desire for _____ [All the sugary carbohydrates—cakes, cookies, donuts, pastries, and sugary cereals—that challenge you] exists sealed in the basket.

Any overwhelming desire for _____ [All forms of chocolate that challenge you] exists sealed in the basket.

Any overwhelming desire for _____ [All kinds of candy that challenge you] exists sealed in the basket.

Any overwhelming desire for _____ [All frozen desserts that challenge you—ice cream and frozen yogurt] exists sealed in the basket.

Any overwhelming desire for _____ [All sodas and sugar-laden drinks, including juice, that challenge you] exists sealed in the basket.

Any overwhelming desire for _____ [All the salty, crunchy snacks that challenge you] exists sealed in the basket.

Any overwhelming desire for _____ [All the kinds of savory carbohydrates—pasta, rice, bread, and pizza—that challenge you] exists sealed in the basket.

Any overwhelming desire for _____ [All the variations of potato that challenge you] exists sealed in the basket

Any overwhelming desire for _____ [All of your favorite fried foods] exists sealed in the basket.

Any overwhelming desire for _____ [All of the cheeses that challenge you] exists sealed in the basket.

Any overwhelming desire for _____ [All of the varieties and variations of nuts that challenge you—nuts to peanut and almond butter] exists sealed in the basket.

Any overwhelming desire for _____ [All of the varieties and brands of fast food that challenge you] exists sealed in the basket.

Any overwhelming desire for _____ [All varieties and kinds of meals that challenge you] exists sealed in the basket.

Any use of food in a hurtful way exists sealed in the basket.

Everything in the basket is in its rightful place.

I cannot miss what I no longer want.

My conscious, logical desires are represented in the basket, so my conscious and subconscious desires are in sync—there is no more ambivalence.

I am in total control of my relationship with food.

[End use of inner voice. Read on.]

So the conscious and subconscious minds are synchronized now. They both want you to be

lean,

strong,

and healthy.

Without feeling deprived, without dieting—in fact, feeling empowered.

Now, I want you to imagine yourself standing next to that basket.

So that you're right there in front of it.

So that the giant balloon is truly looming over you.

You're seeing it.

You're looking up at it.

It's towering over you.

Know that the basket and the balloon hold everything that blocks you from realizing your potential.

Look up and see the field.

See the wide-open potential that lies before you.

Now bring your attention back to the basket.

See the four sandbags.

One draped over each of the four sides of the basket.

They are the only things holding this basket and all your struggles in place.

See that you have the power and strength to move them.

To push them to the ground.

To release your struggle.

The release of this basket is the end of the struggle.

Your freedom, health, and well-being are waiting for you.

Now imagine yourself pushing the first sandbag off the edge of the basket.

See the basket and balloon shift.

Move to another side of the basket and push another sandbag off.

The basket is now pulling up, almost free.

Move to another sandbag. Push the third bag off.

The basket is lifting off.

Run to the final side of the basket.

Release the sandbag.

See the balloon lift off.

Float up.

Carrying away the struggle with it.

It is above the trees now.

It is getting higher and higher.

Floating away beyond the edge of the field.

Watch it go.

See it getting smaller and smaller.

It is now only a speck on the horizon.

And then,

it is gone.

You can no longer see it.

How can something you can no longer see have any control over you?

It can't.

The basket with all that it contains is completely powerless over you.

It is gone.

You cannot see it.

The struggle is in its proper place. There is no ambivalence about this. It has been eradicated from your life.

You have reframed your relationship to food.

You have taken control of your life.

Now, see yourself taking your experience to the next logical level.

Picture yourself

lean,

strong,

and healthy.

Free of the balloon and all that it represents.

Feel and see how good that feels.

You have that entire field to yourself.

Jump around.

Dance.

Sing.

Feel the freedom from the burden.

Feel empowered. Feel in control of food.

You have not only contained the struggle, you have let it go.

And as you continue to enjoy your freedom, repeat this phrase in your inner voice: "_____." [Use your Anchor Statement here.]

Now that you're past your struggle, know that the balloon and all your food issues are behind you.

Every time you reexperience this metaphor of a balloon floating away, the subconscious mind knows exactly what it means.

The struggle is over. You're more free of it with every repetition of the balloon floating away.

The phrase "_____" [Use your Anchor Statement here.] *will forever be linked to the freedom, the fact that you can walk past any old nemesis with ease.*

The struggle is gone. It has floated away.

Anytime you use the phrase "_____"
[Use your Anchor Statement here.] *you are reminding the subconscious mind that you are in control of what, when, where, why, and how much you eat.*

So the phrase and the metaphor of freeing the balloon are one and the same.

The phrase becomes a conditioned response.

Each time you use the phrase, it will trigger an automatic reflex, the instinct to make a healthy choice for mind and body.

This picture of the balloon floating away matches your conscious desire to be free of the struggle and be

lean,

strong,

and healthy.

Your conscious and subconscious minds are in agreement.

You are free of ambivalence.

Your conscious desire to be

lean,

strong,

and healthy

is reflected by your subconscious response to produce this healthy desire.

Every time you use the phrase "_____"
[Use your Anchor Statement here.] *you want to make the healthy choice for mind and body.*

To become and remain lean, strong, and healthy.

Repeat each of the following phrases in your inner voice:

_____. [Use your Anchor Statement here.]

I feel full and satisfied with moderate portions at meals.

Food is fuel for health and well-being.

If there's no need to refuel, then there's no desire for eating.

I refuel only when there's a physiological need.

I am completely indifferent to _____. [All cakes, cookies, donuts, and pastries that challenged you.] I can bypass this/them anytime.

I am completely indifferent to _____. [All forms of chocolate that challenged you.] I can bypass this/them anytime.

I am completely indifferent to _____. [All kinds of candy that challenged you.] I can bypass this/them anytime.

I am completely indifferent to _____. [All frozen treats that challenged you—ice cream and frozen yogurt.] I can bypass this/them anytime.

I am completely indifferent to _____. [All sugary cereals that challenged you.] I can bypass this/them anytime.

I am completely indifferent to _____. [All sodas and sugary drinks, including juice, that challenged you.] I can bypass this/them anytime.

I am completely indifferent to _____. [All the salty, crunchy snacks that challenged you.] I can bypass this/them anytime.

I am completely indifferent to _____. [All the kinds of pasta, pizza, and bread that challenged you.] I can bypass this/them anytime.

I am completely indifferent to _____. [All the variations of potato that challenged you.] I can bypass this/them anytime.

I am completely indifferent to _____. [All the favorite fried foods that challenged you.] I can bypass this/them anytime.

I am completely indifferent to _____. [All the cheeses that challenged you.] I can bypass this/them anytime.

I am completely indifferent to _____. [All the varieties and variations of nuts that challenged you—nuts to peanut and almond butter.] I can bypass this/them anytime.

I am completely indifferent to _____. [All the varieties and brands of fast food that challenged you.] I can bypass this/them anytime.

I reject using food in a hurtful way.

Because I care for my mind and body as I would care for any precious life.

I am a precious life and I use food accordingly.

I would no sooner use food to hurt myself than use it to hurt any innocent life.

I cannot miss what I no longer desire.

I am empowered over food. Never deprived of it.

The only substitute I need is the phrase
"_____." [Use your Anchor Statement here.]

The phrase and my healthy relationship with food are one and the same.

The phrase represents the healthy, empowering use of food.

The phrase becomes more effective every day, with every use of it.

The phrase helps me feel comfortable from within, positive and energized.

The phrase helps me become and remain lean, strong, and healthy.

[Note: End of using the inner voice. The following text is a narrative for you to read and then listen to.]

Now, picture yourself free of the struggle.

Feel the strength you have.

Feel how good it feels to have eliminated the struggle, to be on a supportive path of health and well-being.

You're on your way to becoming and remaining

lean,

strong,

and healthy.

Picture yourself in the field looking

lean,

strong,

and healthy.

Feeling unencumbered. Unblocked.

Each time you experience this, you put the struggle further and further behind you.

You are closer to being healthy, happy, joyous, and free.

[Pause]

Now I want you to picture yourself walking to the end of the field.

When you arrive, see a path.

Now really see that path.

This is the path to health and well-being.

Let the path stand out.

Give it a color.

Give it a texture.

Picture it raised so that it is slightly above the level of the ground you are standing on.

The path is still secure, but it is on a higher plane.

Step up onto this path.

This is the path that leads to your health and well-being.

It is never-ending.

Start walking.

Give the path a scent.

Inhale the sweetness.

Picture yourself being on a higher plane.

Caring for yourself.

See yourself going through your day choosing the healthy foods you have identified.

Choosing _____ instead of _____.

Choosing _____ instead of _____.

Eating _____. [Insert a healthy food from your New Pantry list in Chapter 8.]

Drinking water.

Picture yourself _____. [Insert exercise activity you chose—for example, walking, swimming, biking.]

You are doing this for your mind. Your body.

You are on a higher level.

The path is forever associated with the phrase
" _____." [Use your Anchor Statement here.] *Regardless of the path others choose, you crave the path that's right for you.*

The color you have given your path is also forever linked to this phrase. So every time you see the color, it will reinforce your new relationship with food.

The path and the phrase are one and the same.

Now picture yourself walking on that path.

Picture yourself moving forward at a healthy pace.

You're lighter.

You're not carrying the weight.

The weight is off you.

The struggle is off you.

You took control of it.

It is gone.

There is nothing blocking you or weighing you down.

You are unblocked, unencumbered.

The field is further and further behind you.

Like anything else, the further you walk away from something, the smaller it gets.

In fact, you have walked so far along this path of health and well-being that you cannot even see the field.

The field is out of sight.

And so is the balloon.

If you were to glance back to look for it, you couldn't even see it with binoculars.

It is gone.

You are making your way on the path of empowerment. Of health and well-being.

The path is always with you and always supporting you.

The path of health and well-being is endless.

Picture it going into the horizon.

Never-ending.

The path is representative of your foundation foods.

The foods that you crave in moderate portions. The path where food is fuel for health, enjoyment, and self-respect.

Lean proteins such as _____. This is/they are represented by the path.

Fruits such as _____. This is/they are represented by the path.

Vegetables such as _____. This is/they are represented by the path.

Whole grains such as _____. This is/they are represented by the path.

Condiments such as _____. This is/they are represented by the path.

Dairy products such as _____. This is/they are represented by the path.

Beverages such as _____. This is/they are represented by the path.

Water.

And other healthy choices that fuel your mind and body in an appropriate way.

Every breath you draw,

every step you take,

brings you closer to optimal health and joy.

Lean,

strong,

and healthy.

As you progress forward, think of all the positive things that come with being on the path of health and well-being.

Self-respect.

Ease.

Contentment.

Joy.

Freedom.

Your loved ones.

Health.

Well-being.

*Feeling good, every day, all day, from within, **not** from an external source such as food.*

Continue to picture these things.

Stay with this picture.

Stay with these feelings of love, ease, and contentment until you fall into a very

[Read slowly]

deep,

sound sleep.

[End of script]

Tuning In

Once you have recorded your script, it is time to tune in and listen to it. Here are the essential guidelines for using your audio recording.

Listen to the recording when you are falling asleep.

You should do whatever you typically do to wind down before you turn out the lights: read, watch TV, take a bath, whatever. Once you are just about ready to drift off to sleep—in bed, teeth brushed, face washed, lights out—put on a pair of headphones and play the recording and let it lull you to sleep. I want you to fall asleep while the recording is still playing. You want to have the volume at a normal level, a degree of sound that is comfortable for your ears—not too loud or too soft so you are strained or straining. Remember, you *want* to drift off to sleep as you are listening. The goal is for the message on the recording to appear almost dreamlike. If you do not fall asleep by the time the recording ends, play it again. Maybe you just weren't sleepy enough to fall asleep the first time around. You will likely fall asleep on the second pass. Remember, the recording is designed to help you fall into the alpha sleep state, but a small number of people are just so used to falling asleep a certain way (such as in a totally quiet room or with the TV on) that using the recording just doesn't do the job. If this is the case for you, then hearing it a third time will not necessarily do the trick. If you are still not asleep after the second play, just fall asleep the way you normally would.

If you wake up in the middle of the night to go to the bathroom, to change position, or just because you are feeling restless, put the recording on again. The more you listen, the stronger the picture will become. In fact, if you have the ability and are so inclined, you can listen to the recording all night. You go through the alpha state about every ninety minutes, so within an eight-hour night of sleep you can introduce this new healthy picture to your subconscious mind five times!

Listen to your recording without disruption.

This is important. This means that you probably don't want to have your dog or cat cuddled up next to you or crawling around on your bed. Nor do you want to be in bed next to a partner who is watching TV or a movie or listening to the radio. Whether you are aware of it or not, this kind of activity will disrupt your process. So if there's a snorer next to you, go to another bedroom or find a couch!

Use headphones.

Most of my clients like using headphones or ear buds to limit external sounds and avoid disruption. Most find that the headphones are comfortable and they just knock them off during the night without even realizing it. However, if falling asleep with headphones or ear buds is uncomfortable in any way, then don't use them. Try a stereo instead. Or try a pillow speaker; it's a small half-dollar-size speaker that just sits on the mattress, right next to your pillow. Remember, comfort is key!

Know that, as you listen, you will not necessarily *feel* anything.

Falling asleep with the recording will feel no different from the thousands of nights you've fallen asleep before you used the recording. The difference is just that your subconscious mind is being influenced by a new bedtime story. You are now simply capitalizing on a natural human experience.

This said, you probably will notice that you are more aware of the step-by-step experience of falling asleep. This is something most people are not conscious of. You will notice how sleep comes over you, how your body feels as it drifts into the alpha state—your muscles relax, the body and mind become still and quiet. It's a wonderful experience of self-awareness.

Other than the fact that the recording will make you more conscious of how your body transitions into the alpha state, most of my clients report that they are able to fall asleep more easily and quickly with every night that they listen. And they also say that the quality of sleep is better. The reason for this is that each time your subconscious mind hears the same story, it becomes more and more mesmerizing, literally hypnotizing you into sleep. Now you know why kids like to be read the same story as they fall asleep every night. The familiarity is simultaneously comforting and mesmerizing. If you tend to have difficulty falling asleep and staying asleep, the recording will probably address this struggle, if not completely correct it.

Know that you cannot listen wrong.

As you listen, the goal is to focus on the words of the recording. But no one—not even monks who have been practicing meditation for forty years—has perfect focus. Everyone's attention drifts now and then, especially the first few nights. If you find yourself losing focus, don't beat yourself up. Just acknowledge that your mind wandered and bring yourself back to the narration. This process of losing focus and refocusing will get easier and easier.

It is also important to remember that the more you hear your recording, the more quickly you'll be falling into alpha sleep. In a matter of a few days, you might be aware of hearing only the first few words of the recording! But don't worry, the recording won't go to waste—the rest of it will speak directly to your subconscious mind. Think of your subconscious as a sponge; it just soaks up what comes in.

Listen every night for a week to ten days.

This is vital to your success. If you want to establish a change in your brain, you need to give it a picture to work with. If you give it only three nights' worth of imagery, then it is working with the bare minimum. If you give it seven to ten nights' worth of imagery, however, then you have a much stronger and clearer image in your subconscious mind.

Use your Anchor Statement.

As I've said, this phrase is your anchor, the direct line to your subconscious mind. It should become your new mantra, and it is critical that it becomes part of your daily life. You should say this phrase to yourself:

- Before eating every meal

- When you have cravings

- When the boss offers you a donut

- While watching TV

- At a game

- Whenever you feel the irrational call of food

The reason I tell you to use this phrase before eating, when you have a craving, or any other time you are drawn to food is that it reminds the subconscious mind of the new picture you are trying to draw. It dials up the new picture so that your conscious desire to be lean, strong, and healthy is aligned with your subconscious food blueprint. When we are in the process of drawing a new picture in the subconscious mind, we need to reinforce it. The use of the Anchor Statement is the conscious reinforcement of your new subconscious association with food.

If you are a very visual person and words do not come easily to you, you can use the image of yourself on your path, looking lean, strong, and healthy, and hold it in your mind *as you say the phrase*. But no matter what you use—as you say the phrase, or see the image—it is vital that you reinforce with repetition.

During the week to ten days, notice the change.

After our first session, so many of my clients ask me, "How will I know if the recording is working?" I say, "Easy. You'll experience and notice the changes in your eating habits and food preferences, and you'll be losing weight. Yet you won't be trying to. You'll just be eating differently."

So after three or four days, notice if there has been a change in your relationship with food. Take a look at your script and review the changes you wanted to make. Are they taking place? Compare your results with your script.

Some people find that they have an immediate response. Others find that it takes a few days. And still others find that the second script, which we will discuss in Chapter 10 and record and use in Chapter 11, does the trick.

Evaluating the Experience

If you have seen a dramatic or significant change, congratulations! That is great news, and now you are ready to move on to Chapter 10 and the second script.

If after a week you have seen little or no change, follow this checklist:

1. Have you listened every night as you fall asleep?

    If not, then listen every night for a week and see what happens.

2. Did you fall asleep as you listened, or were you awake when the recording was done?

    If you were still awake after the recording was finished and you tried listening more than once, you may have been listening to it too early. If so, try listening a bit later in the evening. Do this for another week and see if there is a difference. Or, as I mentioned, a small number of people can never fall asleep with the tape, so they must listen and then do whatever it is they need to do to fall asleep. This is just as effective, but the results may take a bit longer.

3. Did you listen without disruption?

    Examine how you were listening. Was there anyone around making noise? Did you feel self-conscious doing this in front of your partner? A group of my clients do feel uncomfortable listening to the tape in front of their partners. They don't want their partner to make fun of them or to hear what the recording is saying. For these folks, I suggest listening to the tape in another room just before they go to sleep and then moving into the shared bedroom. In fact, I've had several clients who have listened to this while lying on their bathroom floors!

4. Have you been using your Anchor Statement?

I can't tell you how many clients don't do this on their first try. Some people simply forget to use it! When they tell me this, I point out that this might mean that they are still ambivalent or scared of really losing weight. Saying this phrase silently to yourself as you begin to eat or to combat a craving is such a simple act and can lead to such great results—why else would you not be using it? So if you did not use the phrase, ask yourself once again why you might want to continue to be in a struggle with food. Think about it. And then start using the Anchor Statement on a regular basis.

5. Did you use the Anchor Statement incorrectly?

This is also unbelievably common. Here are the three most frequent ways that people misuse their Anchor Statements:

- They paraphrase.
  The majority of people misuse their Anchor Statement by paraphrasing. For example, if their Anchor Statement is "I control food. Food cannot control me," they might say something like, "Food does not control me." As we have discussed again and again, the subconscious mind is literal: It only responds as it was directed to respond. If you are paraphrasing, you are not connecting yourself to the exact phrase and the new blueprint your script presented to your subconscious mind. In other words, this discrepancy makes it harder for you to make a direct connection to the new subconscious picture you are trying to tap into and reinforce.

- They use the phrase in the middle of a meal or a binge.
  Saying the phrase at the beginning of a meal or when you have a craving sets the tone and healthy picture you want to

have so that you can respond to the food or craving with your conscious and subconscious desires aligned. Saying the phrase in the middle of a meal or binge is less effective. Of course, if on one or two occasions you have forgotten to use the phrase and remember as you are in the middle of snacking, binging, or just eating a meal, by all means use the phrase. It can only help.

- They make the ultimate Freudian slip.

    Finally, there is a small group of people—5 to 10 percent—who make a Freudian slip and say to themselves, "I cannot control food. Food controls me." You can imagine what kind of response this gets! So listen to what you are saying to yourself. Is it really, "I control food. Food cannot control me"?

If after going through this checklist, you found that you have not been following directions, try listening and following all the directions for another week. See what happens. If there is a response after your second try, this is terrific! Move on to Chapter 10 and the second script.

If you have been doing everything right and feel that you have listened to your recording correctly but are still seeing no response, do not despair. It might be that your subconscious mind is just not receptive to this first script. If this is the case, chances are your subconscious mind will be incredibly responsive to the second script, in the same way that some people do better with aspirin, while others like the effect of acetaminophen. So turn the page and let's move on!

Script II: Writing Your Future

Chapter Ten

Life must be understood backwards;
but ... it must be lived forward.

—Søren Kierkegaard

In the course of reading this book, you have spent most of your time so far reflecting and looking backward to understand why, how, and where you were with your struggle with food. In the first script, we began to shift our focus to the future, looking forward, by introducing a new way of living and relating to food. In this chapter and from here on out, the focus of this book—and I hope of your life— is about moving forward, evolving, growing, and realizing your true potential. There is no more struggle, only a life to be lived.

But what I have often found is that while people can often picture themselves lean, strong, and healthy, they cannot see the kind of life— particularly the details of the life—that leads them to that ideal body or dress size. As you have learned, so much of medical hypnosis is about using the power of your imagination to heal. And as I described in Chapter 3, the second script is mostly about coloring in the newly sketched picture of a healthy relationship with food that the first script outlined.

As you know, my clients typically see me for two medical hypnosis sessions. The second session takes place about a week after the first. (Has it been a week to ten days since you began listening to Script I? If so, keep reading. If not, give yourself at least seven days.)

In this second session, the client and I explore what has changed and what hasn't. We do this so that we can identify and define what the client's subconscious mind needs to hear. With most clients, I have found that the behaviors—snacking, craving, overeating, nocturnal binging—often change within this first week and that many of the "gotta have it" foods become "indifferent" foods, but usually one or two foods still tug at the person and hold them back. The reason? Deeper relationships and neuropathways are harder to break and rewire. In this chapter, we will look at what foods and habits have dissipated and those that have not, and then find the appropriate language for the second script that will break these extra-strong neuropathways down. We will also find language that will help you plan your future relationship with food in greater detail.

Unlike the first script, which operates like a movie trailer, telling the subconscious mind that something is coming and giving it a taste of what it will see, the second script relies on neurolinguistic programming, which, through repetition, shows the subconscious mind the entire movie—the full picture of you looking lean, strong, and healthy. Over time, this picture becomes your reality. Basically, the second script is a long-term dress rehearsal for how your life will unfold from here.

The first thing I want you to do is to read the second script so that you have an idea of what I am looking for when I say that you will rehearse your day. Then we will get to the work of nailing down the issues you still need to erase and the details you want to bring to your days ahead.

The Second Script

Once again, I will talk you through reading and writing a draft of the script so that you become familiar with it and understand how the language draws a picture in the subconscious mind. The first thing you might notice is that this script is much shorter than the first. This is because we are only looking forward. This script does not stop and address the past or a struggle. Essentially, this script is a guided meditation that helps you to rehearse and visualize moving through the day ahead, making healthy choices for your mind and body. In fact, I use a very similar script when I work with athletes and performers to help them break through barriers and play or perform at a higher level.

As with all medical hypnosis scripts, the first thing we begin with is the standard induction, which, as you now know from experience, relaxes you and encourages the brain and body to slow down to the alpha state. I am not including the induction in my explanation of the second script, as you already know it, understand it, and don't need to review it.

Finally, please note that all the sections that are in italics are standard, unchangeable areas of the script. As with Chapter 8, my play-by-play notes to you are written in bold. Once again, if you would like to make a copy rather than work with the book, please do so.

Part I

The Induction

[*Note:* The induction is the same as the one you used in your first script and is included in the version of the second script you will be recording, which comes later in this chapter.]

The Rehearsal

This is the section of the script where you begin to visualize your day. Over the years, I have found that using the metaphor of watching a movie is the easiest way for people to imagine seeing themselves and their day ahead. Remember, the imagination is our movie screen in the mind and the brain reacts to what plays on this screen, real or imagined. Moreover, the act of seeing yourself up on the big screen and larger than life reinforces the idea that, like so many film stars in their roles, you are important and on a lifelong endeavor. But of course I want all my clients to have the red carpet treatment, so I give them their own private screening room. Here it is.

Picture yourself lean, strong, and healthy, walking into an empty private screening room.

The room is the perfect temperature. Not too hot or too cold.

The screening room is dimly lit, with just floor lights illuminating your path.

The walls are covered in a soft, plush fabric.

There are several large and luxurious-looking chairs.

Picture yourself choosing one, walking to the chair, and sitting down.

Notice that it is the most comfortable chair you can imagine.

Every part of your body is supported.

The fabric feels good against your skin.

Your arms, legs, and head relax into the softness and support of the chair.

See yourself in the chair.

You are

lean,

strong,

and healthy.

Now look up at the giant movie screen in front of you.

It is huge, towering over you.

You can see that whatever is going to play on this screen is going to be larger than life.

Know that the movie you are about to watch is going to go exactly as you want it to.

You are in control.

And every time you see this movie, you are having an experience that is a dress rehearsal for how you want to experience yourself and the world around you.

You are the director.

You are the producer.

You are the star.

You are the entire focus of this movie.

Now notice the remote control sitting next to you.

Pick it up.

It has one button that says, "Start my movie."

Picture yourself pressing the button.

Start the movie.

Imagine the light from the projector coming over your shoulder, cutting through the darkness.

Projecting onto and lighting up the screen.

The movie begins with the number 10 in the middle of the screen. The 10 becomes a 9. The 9 turns to an 8. 7 . . . 6 . . . 5 . . . more focused . . . 4 . . . relaxed . . . 3 . . . 2 . . . 1 . . . see the 1 fade away.

"_____." [Your Anchor Statement here.]

The movie continues with the phrase
"_____" [Your Anchor Statement here] *in big bold letters moving across the center of the screen.*

As you watch this, repeat the phrase to yourself, using your inner voice.

Now picture the phrase dropping down to the bottom of the screen so that it rests there like a caption.

And let it remain there so that every frame of the film you will see will have this caption: "_____." [Your Anchor Statement here] *This phrase and every scene of the movie are interrelated.*

Now, I want you to imagine the movie progressing with each of the following phrases appearing, one at a time, at the center of the screen.

After you read the phrase, repeat the phrase using your inner voice:

I am lean, strong, and healthy.

I know the path I'm on and it's the right path for me.

I am free of the struggle with food and weight.

I am empowered over food. Never in a struggle with it.

I am a precious life and I care for my mind and body accordingly.

We will talk about this next section on page 193. But for now, know that this is the section where you will include the unhealthy behaviors that you still occasionally indulge in or succumb to. For instance, if you are a stress eater, you might say, "I reject the notion of using food as a way of relieving stress." As with all of the fill-in-the-blank sections, I've given you a set amount of statements, but if this is not enough or too much, please tailor the script to your needs. Take however much space you need. Say what you need to say.

I reject the notion of _____.

Every day.

I reject the notion of _____.

Every day.

I reject the notion of _____.

Every day.

I reject the notion of _____.

Every day.

I reject the notion of _____.

Every day.

Everyday I have choices to make and I choose self-respect.

I have accomplished extraordinary things and I can accomplish this.

Food is fuel for health and well-being.

I crave healthy foods and eat in moderation.

This next section is the actual rehearsal of the day ahead. This is perhaps the most important part of the entire medical hypnosis process. This is

where, with repetition, you will change your mind, which will, in turn, change your life. Proceed with enthusiasm!

Now, with the phrase "_____"
[Your Anchor Statement here] *at the bottom of the screen, I want you to imagine that the movie continues.*

Picture yourself waking up tomorrow morning after a wonderful night's sleep.

You feel rested, healthy, alive, even joyous.

Now see yourself getting out of bed, swinging your legs over the side, sitting on the edge of your bed.

You are

lean,

strong,

and healthy.

And right there on the floor, just below your feet, is the path of health and well-being, where you are lean, strong, and healthy.

You know the color of the path.

See the color.

See the texture.

The path is glowing, radiating comfort.

Notice once again how it is just above the surface of the floor, yet it is still stable and supportive of you.

It is on a higher plane, as you are on a higher plane.

See yourself making the choice to slip off the bed and step onto the path.

You choose the path because it will always support you.

Because it is the path of health and well-being, self-respect and empowerment.

It is the journey you were meant to take and make.

Every step you take.

Every breath you take.

All day.

Every day.

And anytime you see the color of the path, know that it is there to remind you of what you want most.

To be

lean,

strong,

and healthy.

There is nothing you want more than to be thin.

And the color reminds you of the key phrase,

"_____." [Your Anchor Statement here.]

The color and the phrase are one and the same.

Now I want you to watch the on-screen rehearsal of the day ahead.

How you will go through your day.

Picture yourself moving along the path.

Looking the way you want to look and feel.

Lean.

Strong.

And healthy.

As you walk down the path, notice that the balloon and all that it contains is nowhere in sight.

It is gone.

Now, picture yourself getting ready for the day, making choices that support your health and well-being.

Picture yourself moving through your day with ease.

This is the section where, while listening, you will visualize yourself bypassing those foods that are still giving you trouble, or not engaging in behavior that is self-destructive or hurtful to you—snacking, binging, overeating. For instance, if chocolate is still challenging you, imagine yourself walking by a box of chocolates, or refusing chocolate when offered it, or not eating chocolate when everyone else is gorging on it. Or if snacking is a real problem for you, see yourself doing a mini meditation exercise and eating a piece of fruit as your midafternoon activity to combat stress and fatigue (which is probably why you are snacking in the afternoon). The idea is to use this section of the script to work on the things that are challenging you. It may be that you picture yourself walking by chocolate for some time and then find that chocolate is no longer a problem, but you do still need to see yourself bypassing bread. In other words, this is an ever-evolving process. Use the daily rehearsal to support you in making healthy decisions for your mind and body.

You are

lean,

strong,

and healthy.

Every decision, interaction, movement you make is about realizing your potential.

See the day ahead.

Picture every detail.

See yourself empowered by the choices you are making.

You are free of ambivalence.

You are in control.

Your conscious and subconscious desires to be

lean,

strong,

and healthy

are one and the same.

You feel full and satisfied with moderate portions at meals.

You know that food is fuel for health and well-being.

If there's no need to refuel, then there's no desire for eating.

You eat only when there's a physiological need.

Notice the choices you are making throughout your day.

Notice what you find yourself gravitating toward.

No matter what you are doing, you are making healthy choices in moderation.

Observe how easy it is to bypass without a second thought the habits and behaviors that you no longer need. Remember, you control this movie, so it goes the way you want it to. This means you can stop and replay any segment of the movie. Use this ability to re-rehearse any habits or beliefs that need attention, such as bypassing any food that at this time draws you in. If there are no such foods in your life now, just notice how you easily pass food by, no struggle, no challenge.

Again, this is where, while listening, you will incorporate those foods that are still giving you trouble. You will see yourself not engaging in that particular behavior or indulging in a particular food. And you will see yourself engaging in healthy activities such as exercise, hanging out with friends, spending time with loved ones, and meditating. Be as specific with your goals as you want to be—being able to run a mile, healthy relationships, fulfilling work.

Feel the ease, comfort, and joy you experience.

You can do anything.

You are accomplishing everything you set out to do.

Maybe even more.

Really see the day ahead.

Fill in every detail.

Know that every time you see this rehearsal, you are blurring the line between the interior rehearsal in your head and the external reality that is your life.

Your positive thoughts are becoming a reality.

Remember, you control the movie.

And it always goes exactly the way you want it to.

You are moving forward on the path.

Making huge progress.

Looking the way you want to look, the way you want others to see you.

Lean.

Strong.

And healthy.

Empowered.

Continue to see your day, your successes,

as you fall

into

a

deep

and sound

sleep.

[End of script II]

––––––––––

Now that you have read through this once or twice, you have a much better idea of the depth and clarity you will need to write your future. Let's look at some ways to make the second script as personal and specific as possible.

What Remains?

The first thing we need to look at and evaluate is your receptivity to the first script.

If you have had a great response to the first script, this is wonderful, and I encourage you to personalize and then record the second script, which reinforces all the healthy behaviors you have begun to see emerge. Likewise, if you have had a good response but are finding that one or two things still need a kick out the door, the second script will give those things the boot. And if you have not had great success and are frustrated with this whole process and are wondering if you should even still be reading this or even hoping that medical hypnosis can do anything for you, I beg you to please stay with me for at least this chapter.

Some people—roughly 25 percent—experience little to no change after the first session (the first script). There are dozens of reasons why this is the case. But no matter what the reason is, a resistance to the first script tells me—and you, if you are experiencing it—that the person's subconscious mind might not be ready or able to let go.

If you are experiencing resistance, it is more than likely that you simply have particularly strong neuropathways for specific foods or unhealthy behaviors. Fortunately, if this is your case, your subconscious mind will respond beautifully to the second script and sessions because the second script is devoted to drawing new neuropathways! The only other type of subconscious resistance is due to a deeper, underlying pathology, and unfortunately we cannot know if this is the case until you try using the second script.

What needs to be kicked out the door?

Returning to your Inventory on page 105, which foods are no longer giving you trouble and what foods are still causing a struggle? Write an **N** for "no problem" next to the foods that you now feel indifferent to. And write a **T** for "trouble" next to the foods that are still challenging. Be sure to include foods that you are not necessarily indulging in but still have an inner dialogue with. For instance, if someone brought donuts or chocolates to work in the last week, were you pulled by them? Did you have more than a taste? Or did you make the decision to not eat, but had to leave the room? Remember the goal of this is to feel completely free from the pull of these foods. You can either refuse them or taste them and be done with them. So with that in mind, go through the list on page 105.

On page 205, I will be asking you to write a practice rehearsal of your day to help you think about how you will visualize your day in your head. This is not something you will record; rather, it is a way for you to think about and understand how you will include these T foods and moments in your day, where you will bypass these T foods and/or see yourself saying, "No, thank you" to someone offering some to you. Over time, this mental practice of saying no to unhealthy foods and yes to healthy ones will become a stronger and stronger reality.

Now let's look at what behaviors have ceased and which ones are still cropping up. Return to the list on page 87, and write an **N** next to the behaviors that have ceased. Write a **T** next to the behaviors that are still giving you trouble.

How many Ns did you have? How many Ts? It is my greatest hope that you will have a plethora of Ns and a few Ts. But no matter how many Ts you have, the second script can handle them. Your awareness of the stubborn habits is the first important step.

As you have learned, a vital part of this process is one of self-evaluation—being curious about the pulls, the cravings, the snacking, the desire to binge that affects your health. The more you become aware of what foods you want, how you want them, and what is going on around you physically and emotionally when these urges emerge, the more you can combat these urges using the second script.

In the section of the script that has the phrase "I reject the notion of _____," fill in all the T behaviors. For instance, if you have trouble with eating when you are bored, you would write in, "I reject the notion of eating out of boredom." Or if you are still standing in front of the sink spooning ice cream into your mouth, you would write, "I reject the notion of eating in front of the sink."

Now that you have addressed the unhealthy foods and behaviors that are still lingering after the first script, it is time to look at the healthy behaviors and actions you want to engage in going forward. The first step is to think about and imagine what your healthy relationship with food will be.

What's a Healthy Relationship with Food Anyway?

If you are anything like most of my clients, you may have no idea (or too many ideas) about what a healthy relationship with food is. Many think of a healthy diet as some kind of program that maybe includes lettuce, tofu, deprivation, and—worst of all—feeling hungry. For the record, none of this is true. You are welcome to eat lettuce and tofu, but they do not automatically translate to a healthy relationship with food. Here is how I explain it to my clients:

A healthy relationship with food is not a diet.

Diets are by definition about cutting things out, deprivation, and having *less* of a relationship with food. Eating in a healthy way that feeds your mind and body means that you *do* have a relationship with food. Unlike other addictions—alcohol, cigarettes, caffeine, sugar, drugs— you cannot just stop eating. If you did, you would die. Instead, you must forge a new kind of interaction. This is why food addictions are so hard to unwind and reprogram. However, this is also why medical hypnosis is so effective—because it is the only method that gets into your subconscious mind and even gives you a shot at changing the relationship on a fundamental level, which is what you need to succeed.

If you are in a healthy relationship with food, you should not feel hungry.

Let me say that again: If you have a healthy relationship with food, you should not feel hungry. If you are feeling a craving, are hungry, or like snacking between meals, then it is often a signal that you are not eating proper meals. In other words, you are not providing your body with enough protein and nutrients to fuel your mind and body.

This next section includes my guidelines for having a healthy relationship with food. You will need to incorporate this information into your life on both the subconscious and conscious levels. For now we will look at how to integrate this healthy picture of you interacting with food in a positive way for your script (the subconscious work). In Chapter 11, we will look at how to support the subconscious picture with conscious action.

The fifteen best ways to create a healthy relationship with food

1. Cook your own food.

Believe it or not, cooking your own meals is the first step to having a healthier relationship with food. It gives you much more control over what you eat, when you eat, how you eat it, how much you eat, the ingredients you use, and the quality of the ingredients.

If you have never cooked before or hate the idea of cooking, I understand. I am no Emeril in the kitchen. This said, having a few basics under my belt—egg whites with fresh herbs, grilled salmon on a bed of mixed greens with a balsamic vinaigrette, roast chicken—gives me much more control.

If you are at the mercy of restaurants and frozen foods, you don't always know what is in the food, the quality of the ingredients, or the amounts. For instance, you may want to include some feta in a Greek salad, but if you go to a diner or have a pre-made Greek salad from the market, the salad will more than likely be loaded with twice as much feta as you really need. Moreover, if you're eating food made by others, you have no idea if you are eating genetically modified vegetables, saturated fats, or hidden sugar (often found in restaurant and store-bought sauces and dressings—even ones that are low-fat). Wouldn't you like to know?

2. When cooking, use recipes and stick to them.

You may enjoy cooking by taste; nonetheless, over the years I have found that recipes generally offer the appropriate and right proportions of the food we're cooking. More often than not, recipes use much less fat (cream, cheese, oil) and starch than we would add were we to be ad-libbing.

Finding and cooking new flavors and foods that will fuel your mind and body is part of developing a new relationship with food. For low-fat and flavorful soup, salad, and vegetable recipes, take a stroll through the vegetarian cookbook section of your local library or bookstore for inspiration. There's a whole world of recipes for you to tap and try.

3. Eat food with flavor.

Eating well does not mean chewing on tasteless food the consistency of sawdust. The tastier the food, the more satisfied you will be. Adding butter and fatty foods such as cheese or cream is not the only way to achieve flavor. Use onions, garlic, citrus, or spices such as cumin, chili powder, or even rosemary to add some zing. You'd be amazed by how good steamed spinach is with a little lemon and garlic on it, or how wonderful a poached chicken breast can be if you throw half an onion, black pepper, and a celery stalk into the poaching water. If you must use some kind of fat for cooking, use olive oil. Again, browse your local library or bookstore cookbook section for inspiration.

4. Make a grocery list *before* going to the grocery store.

Having a grocery list is one conscious way of making sure you gravitate toward the right foods. Walking into a grocery store with a list gives you a game plan, a map to follow. To get started, refer to the list I gave you on pages 122 to 124 in Chapter 8. You should always include low-fat dairy, whole grains, lean protein, berries, and vegetables. It is also smart to pick up a few foods that you can take on the go:

A low-carb, low-sugar, low-fat protein drink that does not need refrigeration

A low-carb, low-sugar, low-fat protein bar that does not need refrigeration

Lean protein—turkey slices, lean roast beef, etc.

Healthy snack foods—carrot sticks, rice cakes, hummus

Hand fruit—apples, pears, citrus

You'll find that if you follow the simple list I've given you, you do not even need to walk down the cookie or snack food aisles!

5. Never go shopping when hungry.

Never, ever go grocery shopping when hungry. This is like asking a thirsty alcoholic to go into a bar for a glass of water. Why tempt yourself unnecessarily?

So when is a good time to go? After breakfast, lunch, or dinner. You will be full, satisfied, and less likely to pull those cookies, snack foods, or other trigger foods off the shelves. If you are an eat-while-you-shop person, eat something healthy—a pear, a protein bar, a rice cake, sliced strawberries.

6. When grocery shopping, read the labels.

You wouldn't take medicine without doing some research, right? So why would you put a food in your body if you didn't know what was in it? When buying food, do your research. Read the labels. This will save you from extra calories, fat, chemicals, and sugar, which in large portions can all lead to disease.

Is the first ingredient sugar? Or, more likely, are the first five ingredients five kinds of sugar? If so, the food is probably not good for you. Can't pronounce half the ingredients or don't even know what they are? Know that they are probably chemicals that are not particularly good for your health or well-being. High sodium levels? The U.S. Food and Drug Administration recommends people have less than 2,400 mgs of sodium per day. This means anything with more than 140 mgs of sodium has high sodium. Not good for you. Twelve food dyes or artificial flavors? Not good for you. "All-natural?" Look and see! They may mean that the five kinds of sugar are all natural. "Diet"? While low in calories and fat, it is probably high in chemicals or salt.

These days, there are plenty of whole-food, organic options. The best rule of thumb is to buy unprocessed and organic. It's better for you and the environment. And while a bit more expensive at the check-out, it's much cheaper than the doctor's bills.

7. When cooking and serving, know what a portion is.

Ask twenty-five people what a serving of chicken looks like and you'll get almost as many answers as people. Everyone has their own distorted idea of what size is when it comes to portioning.

Here is my definition of proper and appropriate portions:

- A portion of protein should be the size of the surface of your fist (palm side up) and about as thick as the distance from the tip of your thumb to the first knuckle.

- If you are a man, a portion of starch (potato or pasta, if you eat these at all) should be about the same size as your fist. If you are a woman, make a fist and make the portion size maybe a third smaller. Remember, a single slice of bread is a portion.

- As for vegetables, you can eat all the vegetables you want (within reason, of course). I recommend that you eat your vegetables steamed, with little or no butter. Turn to the huge assortment of spices for flavoring.

- When it comes to fruit, choose types low in carbohydrates. This includes berries, apples, and pears. But, of course, know that eating a peach or a piece of melon is completely fine. Carbohydrate-rich fruits are always a much better treat for your mind and body than carbohydrate-rich foods such as cookies or potato chips.

8. Eat three meals a day that will fuel your mind and body.

Do you ever feel like eating two hours after a meal—particularly after breakfast or lunch? Most people think that healthy eating means eating a bowl of fruit for breakfast, a plain salad for lunch, five almonds at three, and a piece of steamed fish for dinner. If you have eaten like this or think healthy eating is this, then it's no wonder you are hungry or associate healthy eating with hunger!

A client recently came into my office after doing her second script and told me that she was really struggling. She said she had been doing beautifully during the day—making healthy choices and not craving foods—but by the time she got home and began to make dinner, she couldn't help herself. She snacked and picked at everything as she cooked. I asked her what she was eating during the day. She told me a light breakfast of a low-carbohydrate cereal and a salad for lunch. I said, "Well, it's no wonder you're hungry! You're starving yourself! A little cereal and a green salad is not enough to fuel a day." Of course, she was making up for this deprivation by grazing before dinner. I told her that she needed to add protein to her breakfast and lunch meals—maybe egg whites in the morning and some steamed or grilled chicken or fish on her salads at lunch. A week later, she called me and said, "Ron! With this new schedule, I have so much energy. I can't believe it!"

Eating three meals a day means eating *three portions* of lean protein and *three portions* of fruit and vegetables. If you eat more of the right foods, then you will eat less of the wrong ones.

9. Eat regularly.

Don't eat breakfast at six in the morning and then make your body wait until three for lunch and wait again until ten for dinner. This is a recipe for hunger and powerful cravings. If you have a crazy day ahead of you, make sure that you are feeding your body lean protein, vegetables, and some fruit every four hours.

The best way to do this is to set mealtimes for yourself. If you are not going to be able to make a particular mealtime, have a protein bar or shake to support your system until you can feed yourself. Which leads me to number 10:

10. Eat well no matter how busy you are.

Nearly everyone I see says they don't have time to eat right. Well, it takes the same time to eat right as it does to eat wrong. So make life really easy and have the following available wherever you might be:

A healthy (read labels) protein drink that does not need refrigeration

A healthy (read labels) protein bar that does not need refrigeration

At home (and at work if you have a refrigerator there) always try to have:

- Lean protein—turkey slices, lean roast beef, etc.

- Healthy snack foods—carrot sticks, rice cakes, hummus

- Hand fruit—apples, pears, citrus

This way, if you are running out the door or into a meeting, you can still grab something that will feed your mind and body, taste good, and not leave you starving later.

11. Make lunch your biggest meal of the day.

The beginning and middle of the day is when you are most active and therefore you need the most fuel, so why not eat to fuel this need? Even if you change nothing else, eating your biggest meal in the middle of the day helps just about every person I see lose weight. Eat a proper breakfast, back it up with a healthy and satisfying lunch, then make dinner a bit lighter. What do you have to do after dinner, anyway? Sit? Read? Watch TV? Sleep? You don't need tons of fuel for that. But you do need fuel for the fifty things you must do between 9 A.M. and 6 P.M. Think of your body as a car. Give it gas when you are using it, not when it is sitting in the garage.

12. When out to lunch or dinner, watch others as they belly up to the trough.

You're out for a nice dinner or a special lunch. Want to instantly make a better choice about what to eat? As you enter the restaurant and while you sit at the table before ordering, take a look around you. How do the other diners look as they eat? What are they eating? How are they eating? Notice who is stuffing themselves. Notice who is not. Really study what people are doing to themselves and ask yourself: "How do I want to look to others if they were to look around and see me eating? Do I want to look like a pig standing at a trough? Or do I want to look like a self-respecting person who cares for my mind and body?"

Another hint: If you know what you want to order, don't look at the menu. Doing so only causes a conditioned response. That is, if you read the description of a really fattening comfort meal, you are likely to experience a craving. And yes, it appears so real to the brain that you can actually feel your stomach growling and your salivary glands going into action in response to the menu description. If you don't have a meal in mind, instead of looking at the menu, ask the wait staff what they have in the way of vegetables, lean protein, or a salad with lean protein. This will give you more than enough to go on.

Another great rule is to not look at the dessert menu. Why should you? It's so much easier not to. I used to peruse dessert menus not at all hungry, completely stuffed. Then I'd see something jump off the page at me. Who needs that? If I don't look, my old blueprint is not triggered or tugged at and I don't care. Try it and see!

13. Don't make three different dinners each night.

Does your family eat in shifts—at five for the one who has theater practice or a tutor at six, six for the other one after she gets home from sports, and eight for you and your partner? This kind of schedule can only lead to snacking and cravings—and it means that you are probably in and out of the kitchen for roughly four or five hours. Not good. You can be around food only so much before temptation and snacking kick in. You're only human!

The solution? Set kitchen hours and make one meal. If members of the family can't make it to the table at the set time, then the rule is that dinner will be in the fridge, oven, or microwave. (*Before you do this, be sure to have a conversation with the family. Make the time of the meal a group decision if the kids are old enough.*) And finally, know that offering your kids one meal rather than catering to their needs and preferences may cause an uproar now but will help to foster healthy eating habits for the future.

14. Exercise.

I know you don't want to hear this, but in addition to all its other benefits, exercise is a wonderful vehicle for helping us develop a healthy relationship with food. Try eating a pizza for lunch and then going for a walk or run in the late afternoon. Your body will hurt. But if you eat a nourishing bowl of steamed vegetables and meat at lunchtime and then go for a walk or run, your body will hurt less, maybe even feel good.

For me and many of my clients, exercise is a great barometer for helping us identify what kind of eating plan is best for our unique bodies. Moreover, if you exercise regularly, it increases your metabolism; is wonderful for your heart, muscles, bones, and mental state; and, most importantly, will teach you what true hunger is!

15. Use my four-step method to combat cravings: stop/anchor/determine/decide.

You have a thought to eat that seemingly comes out of nowhere. Before eating anything:

Stop. Don't react so fast and just start eating, as you have done in the past.

Anchor. Use your Anchor Statement.

Determine. Ask yourself, "What's the reason for the desire? Is it *true* hunger?" If it is, a small, healthy snack is in order. "Or is it an emotional craving/reaction?" If so, to what? To whom?

Decide. If there is no true need to eat, ask yourself this: "Am I going to do what I've always done in this situation—eat when there's no real need for food—or am I going to take the healthy, self-respecting action and address the underlying issue (anger, stress, hurt, etc.) at hand?" By getting to the real reason for the craving and addressing it, you will begin to rewire your brain not to expect the same old behavior (the reward of food) but to expect a new behavior (knowing what you really want and giving that to yourself).

Now I've given you my fifteen rules for establishing a healthy relationship with food. In the next section, I'm going to ask you to visualize a day ahead. Are there any suggestions in these rules that you can apply to the way you live and work right now? Go through the following questions and answer honestly.

Can you cook for yourself?

Do you want to?

Can you begin to use less fat and more spices?

Will you buy some cookbooks to help inspire you?

Will you make a grocery list that you can stick to?

When will you grocery shop?

Will you make sure that you are not hungry as you walk into the store or that you have something with you to satisfy the hunger in a healthy way?

Will you read the labels?

Will you look at the portions you are serving?

Will you eat three meals a day?

Will you make a schedule so that you can eat regularly?

If your life does not allow for a regular eating schedule, will you allow for this by having healthy foods around to eat?

Will you make lunch your biggest meal of the day?

Will you eat less at night?

If restaurants are a huge trigger for you, what will you do to support your conscious desire to be lean, strong, and healthy?

Will you get out of the multiple-dinner habit even if it means the kids must zap their food?

Will you make time to exercise?

Will you use your Anchor Statement or do a mini meditation if you feel a craving?

Will you stop/anchor/determine/decide?

Will you be proactive with your conscious desire and new subconscious desire to be lean, strong, and healthy?

Dream Your Day

Because so much of the second script relies on the power of your imagination and your ability to "see" a healthy life for yourself, I want you to take a moment and give yourself a chance to practice imagining your dream day.

Set aside an hour or so to write down a dream day scenario. This does not mean I want you to make up a completely unrealistic fantasy life that you'd like to lead. It means I want you to reimagine the life you have where you are lean, strong, and healthy and have found a positive way to interact with food. Be as specific as possible. See the color of your bedroom. See your healthy, fit body. Describe it. See your meals. Describe them. Use the following questions to help inspire and draw your day:

What does the day look like?

What is the weather like?

What time do you get up?

What do you do next?

Do you exercise?

Do you meditate?

Do you shower or eat first?

Will you use your Anchor Statement throughout the day?

What are you wearing?

How does your body look in clothes?

Do you make time to eat?

Do you drive to work? Take the train? The bus?

How do you feel on your way to work?

How do you feel walking into your office?

What does it look like?

How do you interact with people?

Does someone offer you coffee or tea or food? Do you accept it?

Will you bypass a T food?

How do you feel sitting down to work?

Do you like what you are doing?

Are you able to focus?

Are you able to laugh when something goes wrong?

What do you do for lunch?

What time do you eat?

What are you eating?

Where are you eating?

How do you feel eating lunch?

Are you eating with someone?

Do you take a walk around the block after eating before heading back to work just to clear your head?

Do you do a mini meditation to alleviate some of the stress that has built up during the morning?

Do you smile when people walk past you?

Do you have a good afternoon?

What do you do to alleviate stress?

How do you handle a late-afternoon craving?

Do you feel engaged?

How are you interacting with your coworkers now?

What time do you go home?

How do you get home?

Is walking home your method of exercise?

Do you go to the gym?

Do you go to the grocery store?

What will you have for dinner?

Will you cook?

Will you cook for yourself, or for yourself and others?

How much time will you spend in the kitchen?

How will you make this an enjoyable experience?

Where will you have dinner?

How will you feel while eating?

Will you clean up or will others do it for you?

What will you do after dinner?

What will you do to get ready for bed?

What will you do before going to sleep?

Will you rehearse your day ahead?

This may seem like a ton of questions, but they are intended to get you started and thinking. You don't need to write a book, but I do want you to get into this. Let yourself go. Really picture the life you want. The more you can see yourself lean, strong, and in a healthy relationship with food, the better chance you have of realizing it.

When you are done, take a deep breath and relax. The next step is to plan a time for yourself to record your second script. When you are ready, move on to Chapter 11.

Recording Script II

Chapter Eleven

As a single footstep will not make a path on the earth,
so a single thought will not make a pathway in the mind.
To make a deep physical path, we walk again and again.
To make a deep mental path, we must think over and over
the kind of thoughts we wish to dominate our lives.

—Henry David Thoreau

You have now listened to the first script and prepared for the second. I hope that you can already see how you have begun to draw a new food blueprint in your mind.

This second CD is the key to permanent weight loss. Neurolinguistic programming can and will make a lasting mark on your life if you let it. You just need to give the process a chance.

How to Record the Second Script

Chapter 10 helped you prepare your second script. Once again, I have provided another copy of the script here without my play-by-play comments. Go ahead and fill in the "I reject the notion of _____" section and your Anchor Statement, and have a sense of what kind of day you will be visualizing, including the T foods you will be bypassing. Once you have done this, it is time for you to record Script II.

As with Script I, all the rules for recording still apply:

- Use a technology that is accessible and easy for you to use.

- Give yourself at least an hour to record the script, doing a few practice sessions before making the final usable recording.

- Record the script in a quiet place.

- Know that it does not have to be perfect. Again, if as you are recording the script you change a word here or there unconsciously or because you have a terrible association with that word or just don't like it, please change it. Or if you find yourself adding imagery to the screening room section of the script, by all means, go ahead. **This said, you must not change the language in the script where you use your inner voice. Nor can you change your Anchor Statement. As you know, this phrase is the foundation of the script and of your recovery.**

Take one last moment to ask yourself, "Have I included everything? Are all the foods and behaviors listed?" If so, then, you are ready to record. As before, remember to breathe!

As with the first script, anything in brackets is an action to be done, not read. For instance, when you see "[Pause]," pause for a moment while reading.

Part I

[Read]

Be sure you're in a comfortable position.

With your eyes closed.

The head and neck supported well.

Ready for sleep.

Remember, do not hesitate or prevent yourself from falling asleep while listening. Remember, the early stage of sleep is the deepest form of the alpha or hypnotic state. So I encourage you to fall asleep while listening.

[Pause]

Place one hand on your lower belly.

The reason for doing this is to be sure that you are breathing from your belly. Not your chest. Not your shoulders. Just the lower abdomen. Feel the belly rising and falling as you breathe. Your chest and shoulders should be relaxed and at ease.

Breathing in this way always helps induce relaxation and sleep.

Take a deep cleansing breath in through your nostrils.

And then a nice slow exhale through your mouth.

Just notice your hand rising and falling with each breath, indicating your belly is doing the work.

Take another deep cleansing breath in through your nostrils.

And a nice slow exhale through your mouth.

And repeat that one more time.

Inhale.

Exhale.

And when you complete this deep breath, continue to breathe in a normal fashion.

Through your nostrils.

If you have trouble breathing through your nostrils, then just breathe through your mouth.

And just continue to breathe normally.

Observe the flow of air coming in and out, while focused on the sound of your voice.

Try to leave the rest of the world on hold. And just be focused on your own words.

[Pause]

To help relax further:

Tense up all the muscles in your forehead.

Squeeze your eyes shut so they're squinched up as tightly closed as possible.

Clench your teeth tightly.

Now tense up all the facial muscles.

Tighten them.

Hold that.

A little tighter.

Tighter.

Tighter.

And relax, letting your facial muscles go.

Breathe.

Inhale.

Exhale.

Good.

Notice how good the facial muscles feel, so relaxed.

Now, be sure your head is supported well. No strain on your neck or back.

Let your head just feel heavy, supported, tension-free, easy.

Now, raise your shoulders toward your ears as if you're trying to touch your earlobes.

Higher.

Higher.

Higher.

And let them drop, like they have weights pressing on them.

Nice and heavy and relaxed.

Let them go.

Inhale.

Exhale.

Good.

Now, I want you to think of yourself as being as relaxed as a rag doll.

In fact, use that image.

Imagine you're looking at a rag doll just slumped in a chair.

Totally effortless.

Completely relaxed.

Imagine being that comfortable and relaxed.

Hold that image and thought in your mind as you continue to relax further.

Now tense up all the muscles in your arms.

Make fists.

Squeeze.

Tighter.

Tighter.

Tighter.

And release.

Relax.

Let those arms just drop and relax, like heavy weights.

Let them feel heavy.

Now bear down on the belly.

Tighten up on the abdominal muscles.

Squeezing.

Tighter.

Tighter.

Tighter.

And relax.

Take a deep breath in through your nose.

And a nice long exhale through your mouth.

Let go of any remaining tension.

Drift and relax.

And finally, tense up all the muscles in your legs, from the buttocks all the way to the toes.

Tense your thighs.

Point your toes. Straight out.

Tense your calves.

Hold that.

Tighter.

Tighter.

Tighter.

And let them drop.

Nice and heavy.

Like logs.

And relax.

Take another deep breath in through your nostrils.

And exhale, letting the breath out through your mouth, nice and slow.

Let it all go.

Notice how the body feels now.

How relaxed.

Like a rag doll.

Notice how slow your breathing has become and how much slower it will be over the next few minutes. Notice how cool the air is on your inhale and how warm it is when you exhale.

Good.

The body has moved into a meditative, profoundly relaxed state and will continue to do so with each breath.

This is known as the alpha state. This is when the subconscious mind is most open and most receptive to the information that comes in. In this case, your newly established relationship with food will be imprinted. You will no longer struggle with food.

Use your imagination now.

Picture everything that is now being described.

Imagine you're at the top of a staircase.

There are ten stairs going down below you.

Picture yourself at the top of the staircase.

See yourself the way you want to look.

Lean.

Strong.

Healthy.

Get a good picture of yourself.

Make sure you see your face as clearly as you can. Know that it is you who looks so great.

See the outline of your body exactly as you want it to be.

Lean.

Strong.

Healthy.

Get a vivid picture in your mind's eye.

This picture is not as a result of a diet or struggle or the feeling of being deprived.

In fact, it is the result of the opposite of feeling deprived.

This picture of you,

lean,

strong,

and healthy,

is a result of a new healthy relationship with food where you are in control.

And free of the struggle.

You feel empowered.

Picture yourself now,

lean,

strong,

and healthy,

at the top of the stairs with this feeling of empowerment and self-respect for your mind and body.

As you hear the counting from ten to one, picture yourself taking a corresponding step down those stairs.

[Read steadily]

Ten.

Nine.

Each step a little more relaxed than before.

Eight.

More focused.

Seven.

Deeper and deeper relaxation.

Six.

Five.

Four.

Three.

Two.

One.

Bottom of the stairs.

Anytime you hear yourself count from ten to one while picturing yourself going down those stairs, you'll enter a deeper, more focused alpha state and become more receptive than the time before.

[End of the induction]

Picture yourself lean, strong, and healthy, walking into an empty private screening room.

The room is the perfect temperature. Not too hot or too cold.

The screening room is dimly lit, with just floor lights illuminating your path.

The walls are covered in a soft, plush fabric.

There are several large and luxurious-looking chairs.

Picture yourself choosing one, walking to the chair, and sitting down.

Notice that it is the most comfortable chair you can imagine.

Every part of your body is supported.

The fabric feels good against your skin.

Your arms, legs, and head relax into the softness and support of the chair.

See yourself in the chair.

You are

lean,

strong,

and healthy.

Now look up at the giant movie screen in front of you.

It is huge, towering over you.

You can see that whatever is going to play on this screen is going to be larger than life.

Know that the movie you are about to watch is going to go exactly as you want it to.

You are in control.

And every time you see this movie, you are having an experience that is a dress rehearsal for how you want to experience yourself and the world around you.

You are the director.

You are the producer.

You are the star.

You are the entire focus of this movie.

Now notice the remote control sitting next to you.

Pick it up.

It has one button that says, "Start my movie."

Picture yourself pressing the button.

Start the movie.

Imagine the light from the projector coming over your shoulder, cutting through the darkness.

Projecting onto and lighting up the screen.

The movie begins with the number 10 in the middle of the screen. The 10 becomes a 9. The 9 turns into an 8. 7 . . . 6 . . . 5 . . . more focused . . . 4 . . . relaxed . . . 3 . . . 2 . . . 1 . . . see the 1 fade away.

"_____." [Your Anchor

Statement here.]

The movie continues with the phrase
"_____." [Your Anchor

Statement here.] *in big bold letters moving across the center of the screen.*

As you watch this, repeat the phrase to yourself, using your inner voice.

Now picture the phrase dropping down to the bottom of the screen so that it rests there like a caption.

And let it remain there so that every frame of the film you will see will have this caption: "_____." [Your Anchor Statement here.]

This phrase and every scene of the movie are interrelated.

Now, I want you to imagine the movie progressing with each of the following phrases appearing, one at a time, at the center of the screen.

After you read the phrase, repeat the phrase using your inner voice:

I am lean, strong, and healthy.

I know the path I'm on and it's the right path for me.

I am free of the struggle with food and weight.

I am empowered over food. Never in a struggle with it.

I am a precious life and I care for my mind and body accordingly.

I reject the notion of _____.

Every day.

I reject the notion of _____.

Every day.

I reject the notion of _____.

Every day.

I reject the notion of _____.

Every day.

I reject the notion of _____.

Every day.

Every day I have choices to make and I choose self-respect.

I have accomplished extraordinary things and I can accomplish this.

Food is fuel for health and well-being.

I crave healthy foods and eat in moderation.

Now, with the phrase "_____" [Your Anchor Statement here] *at the bottom of the screen, I want you to imagine that the movie continues.*

Picture yourself waking up tomorrow morning after a wonderful night's sleep.

You feel rested, healthy, alive, even joyous.

Now see yourself getting out of bed, swinging your legs over the side, sitting on the edge of your bed.

You are

lean,

strong,

and healthy.

And right there on the floor, just below your feet, is the path of health and well-being, where you are lean, strong, and healthy.

You know the color of the path.

See the color.

See the texture.

The path is glowing, radiating comfort.

Notice once again how it is just above the surface of the floor, yet it is still stable and supportive of you.

It is on a higher plane, as you are on a higher plane.

See yourself making the choice to slip off the bed and step onto the path.

You choose the path because it will always support you.

Because it is the path of health and well-being, self-respect, and empowerment.

It is the journey you were meant to take and make.

Every step you take.

Every breath you take.

All day.

Every day.

And anytime you see the color of the path, know that it is there to remind you of what you want most.

To be

lean,

strong,

and healthy.

There is nothing you want more than to be thin.

And the color reminds you of the key phrase,

"_____." [Your Anchor Statement here.]

The color and the phrase are one and the same.

Now I want you to watch the on-screen rehearsal of the day ahead.

How you will go through your day.

Picture yourself moving along the path.

Looking the way you want to look and feel.

Lean.

Strong.

And healthy.

As you walk down the path, notice that the balloon and all that it contains is nowhere in sight.

It is gone.

Now, picture yourself getting ready for the day, making choices that support your health and well-being.

Picture yourself moving through your day with ease.

You are

lean,

strong,

and healthy.

Every decision, interaction, movement you make is about realizing your potential.

See the day ahead.

Picture every detail.

See yourself empowered by the choices you are making.

You are free of ambivalence.

You are in control.

Your conscious and subconscious desires to be

lean,

strong,

and healthy

are one and the same.

You feel full and satisfied with moderate portions at meals.

You know that food is fuel for health and well-being.

If there's no need to refuel, then there's no desire for eating.

You eat only when there's a physiological need.

Notice the choices you are making throughout your day.

Notice what you find yourself gravitating toward.

No matter what you are doing, you are making healthy choices in moderation.

Observe how easy it is to bypass without a second thought the habits and behaviors that you no longer need. Remember, you control this movie, so it goes the way you want it to. This means you can stop and replay any segment of the movie. Use this ability to re-rehearse any habits or beliefs that need attention, such as bypassing any food that at this time draws you in. If there are no such foods in your life now, just notice how you easily pass food by, no struggle, no challenge.

Feel the ease, comfort, and joy you experience.

You can do anything.

You are accomplishing everything you set out to do.

Maybe even more.

Really see the day ahead.

Fill in every detail.

Know that every time you see this rehearsal, you are blurring the line between the interior rehearsal in your head and the external reality that is your life.

Your positive thoughts are becoming a reality.

Remember, you control the movie.

And it always goes exactly the way you want it to.

You are moving forward on the path.

Making huge progress.

Looking the way you want to look, the way you want others to see you.

Lean.

Strong.

And healthy.

Empowered.

Continue to see your day, your successes,

as you fall

into

a

deep

and sound

sleep.

[End of script II]

How to Listen to the Second Script

The same rules for listening to the first script still apply when listening to the second:

- Listen to the recording when you are falling asleep.

- Listen to your recording without disruption.

- Use headphones (if you can).

- Know that as you listen, you will not necessarily *feel* anything.

- Know that you cannot listen wrong.

- Continue to use your Anchor Statement. Remember, it is extremely important that you say this phrase to yourself through-out the day:

  o Before eating every meal

  o If you have cravings

  o When the boss offers you a donut

  o While watching TV

  o At a game

  o Whenever you feel the irrational call of food

Again, if you are a very visual person and words do not come easily to you, you can use the image of yourself on your path, looking lean, strong, and healthy, instead of the phrase. But no matter what you use—as you say the phrase or see the image—it is vital that you use one method.

- While listening, be sure to use the rehearsal part as a place where you see yourself making healthy choices, bypassing foods and behaviors that you once indulged and engaged in. Remem-ber, the subconscious is what needs rehearsal—your conscious self has always known what's best for you.

- Listen every night for two weeks, then listen every other night until you reach your goal weight. Once you reach your goal weight, you should listen to it once a week to keep the weight off for life.

- Recall the further changes you wanted to make. Are they taking place? Again, compare your results with your script. After the first two weeks, you can modify the rehearsal section of the script as necessary to address new problems that crop up.

- After you've listened for two full weeks, you can move on to Chapter 12, where you will find my prescriptions for every kind of response, including the small percentage of those who have not seen results thus far.

Conscious Contact

While you spend the next two weeks building a strong foundation for a new food blueprint using the second script, you must also work on your new relationship with food on the conscious level. You already have a conscious desire to be lean, strong, and healthy, but you also need to become aware of how you are supporting this conscious desire in concrete ways. Here are some tips for conscious actions you can take to support the new subconscious picture:

1. Follow my prescriptions for a healthy relationship with food in Chapter 10: Cook your own food, grocery shop with a healthy list, eat regularly—you get the idea.

2. Have a personal cheerleading squad. Tell a few friends about what you are doing, and ask them to support you, encourage you, cheer for you.

3. Use your Anchor Statement. If you have a craving, use it. Use it before you eat. Use it if you are upset. It is your rock. Lean on it. It, along with a few deep breaths or a mini meditation, will always tell you if a hunger feeling is a fact or just a feeling.

4. Be curious. If you have a craving, if you want to snack, or even if you suddenly find yourself with your hand already in the bag or around the fork, don't be upset by it. Get curious. Stop. Take a breath. And then take a moment to look at what led to this craving or eating. What happened? What triggered your

response? Ask yourself what you can do next time to avoid this event. Think of yourself as both scientist and subject.

5. Don't dwell. If something bad happens—someone is rude to you, your boss yells at you, you binge—don't make it worse by dwelling on it. We frequently "awfulize" these events, which means that we make them worse by adding other bad events or feelings onto them. This can make a strong argument for emotional eating in our irrational subconscious minds. For instance, if the boss yells at you about a mishandled interaction with a client, you might go on to add several layers to this: the feeling that you are a terrible person, that you will be fired, that when you are fired you will not be able to pay the bills and then you will be starving. Then you might find yourself thinking, "Food would be nice right about now." See how awful you can make it and how it can only lead you to food? If something unpleasant does happen to you, don't make it worse. Just feel the uncomfortable feeling and let it go.

6. Pause before listening to your head. If your brain is still screaming for you to eat everything on your plate, eat half and immediately take the plate to the kitchen. Just because your head is telling you something doesn't mean that you have to respond to it. Obey your own healthy voice. Take a breath before reacting to a message from your brain.

7. Embrace change. Change your routine. Change your route to work. Change the way you greet your coworkers. Change the way you make your bed. Change for the sake of change, because that is what this process is about. These small gestures support the change that is happening in your subconscious mind.

8. Do something that makes you feel good and is an act of self-love. If you are a person who ate out of deprivation or for love, you need to find activities that bring the feeling of fortune and bounty into your life. This may mean spending time with friends, exercising, or treating yourself to a relaxing massage.

9. When eating, be present in the experience. Don't read or watch TV. Take your time. Chew your food. Experience the taste of it. If you do this, you will find yourself incredibly satisfied at the end of every meal.

10. Don't lie to yourself. If you are not listening to your CD or you are sneaking extra food, admit it. The unfortunate reality of having a food addiction is that everyone knows or will soon know. They can or will see it. If you are eating, it will show. At this stage, the reason you are eating is probably that you are not listening to your CD. So if you are not listening, ask yourself why not.

As you move through the next two weeks, listening to your CD at night, try to incorporate some or all of these principles into your life. My guess is that they will make as much of a difference as the script will. Consciously supporting the new subconscious picture can only lead to a faster and more fully realized shift in your relationship with food.

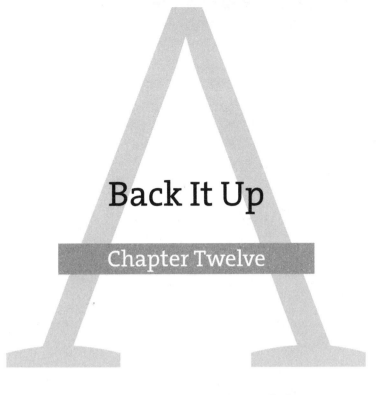

Back It Up

Chapter Twelve

The most important thing to do is really listen.

—Itzhak Perlman

More often than not, two weeks after the second session, a client will call or e-mail to report something like, "I am in *complete control* of my eating, and I am finding the whole process *totally effortless!*"

If a client has not seen a total turnaround, then I hear either: "It's kind of working, but there are still some foods that I can't tackle" or "This was a disaster. I give up." This is rare, of course.

No matter what your answer is, this chapter is here to help you evaluate where you are in this process. It will help you refine and encourage the changes you have seen or help you explore why this process may not have worked for you thus far.

Where Are You in This Process?

As with the first script, some people find that they have an immediate response to the second script and it boosts their newfound immunity to the foods they used to struggle with. If you can identify with this and feel you are doing well, you can either read on or skip ahead to page 237, where I will talk about what to do next and how to continue to support your journey to health and weight loss. But for those of you who are struggling, please read on. There are still many techniques and approaches to be tried.

If you have seen no change to a moderate amount of change with the second script, run through this checklist first before delving into the deeper issues and the prescriptions that follow:

1. Have you listened to the second script every night as you fall asleep?

    If not, then commit to listening every night for two weeks and see what happens.

2. Did you fall asleep as you listened or were you awake when the recording was done?

    If you were still awake after the recording was finished and tried listening more than once, you may have been listening to it too early. If so, try listening a bit later in the evening. Do this for another week and see if there is a difference. Or, as I mentioned, a small percentage of people can never fall asleep with the tape, so they must listen and then do whatever it is they need to do to fall asleep.

3. Did you listen without disruption?

    Was there anyone around making noise? Did you feel self-conscious doing this in front of your partner? As I said in Chapter 9, some of my clients feel uncomfortable listening to the tape in front of their partner. Maybe the first week or so of listening was not an issue for the two of you but now it is? If so, I suggest listening to the tape in another room just before you go to sleep and then moving into the shared bedroom. Or go to page 232 and find out about listening to your recording in the morning, which is an alternative for those who cannot get around family distractions and/or partner issues.

4. Did you use your Anchor Statement?

    Once again, I can't tell you how many clients don't use their Anchor Statement or use it with the first script and don't use it with the second script. If you did not use the phrase, or if you used it, saw some success, and then stopped using it, ask yourself, "Why might I want to continue to be in a struggle with food?" Think about it.

5. Did you use your Anchor Statement correctly?

    After a few weeks, have you begun to paraphrase? Or do you use it in the middle of a meal or binge instead of at the beginning to set the tone? Or did you accidentally twist the phrase around?

Finally, before we dive into the more confounding issues that can prevent the subconscious mind from accepting or embracing change fully, you should know that sometimes it takes the subconscious mind more than a few weeks to accept the suggested change. More often than not, this is because the neuropathway is particularly fortified by years and years of behavior. For instance, if you have used pretzels and chips to alleviate stress and upset for twenty years, then it is going to take a bit of time to break this pattern.

Exercise for Non-Listening Nights

If you have seen a moderate change, I suggest that you use the non-listening nights as a time to picture in your mind's eye the new relationship you want to have with a particular food. As you fall asleep, picture the new relationship you want to have with the few key foods that are still holding you back. You don't need to make a tape or write a script. Just spend a few minutes picturing yourself feeling indifferent to that food—passing it without a thought, saying "No, thank you" when it is offered to you, not grabbing it when you are stressed and instead taking a few deep breaths and saying your Anchor Statement. As with the rehearsal that you are doing with the recording, this small exercise of seeing yourself in control of the troublesome foods will become reality with repetition. Soon you will find that you have disconnected the wiring and are truly free of the foods and behaviors that seemed as though they had immense strength. Repetition of the desired relationship with food is your key to success.

Practice Makes Picture Perfect

The other thing that can cause someone to have only a moderate response with the second script is that the idea of rehearsing the upcoming day is hard for the subconscious and conscious minds to get used to. Picturing something and imagining it happening may be such a foreign concept for your mind that it may take a bit of time for your "fantasy muscle" to be strong enough to be effective.

If you have seen a moderate change after the first two weeks, give yourself another week to ten days to strengthen your fantasy muscle and use the non-listening-nights exercise as a way to reframe the particular foods that are still dogging you. More often than not, time and this exercise give clients who have had a moderate response to the second script a boost. If it does, then you can skip ahead to page 237. If it does not, then let's go through my next level of evaluation to see if we can determine what is preventing your subconscious mind from accepting the idea of change.

Troubleshooting: Phase I

If you have been following the recommended procedures, using your Anchor Statement correctly, have listened to the second script properly for at least two weeks, and tried the non-listening-nights exercise, but still are not having much success, then let's dig in and figure out why your subconscious mind is so ferociously resisting change. The first layer of resistance includes these possibilities:

- Your subconscious mind likes the first script better.

- You are falling asleep too fast, too soundly.

- You don't have enough to do in your day-to-day life.

- You have too much to do in your day-to-day life.

You saw results with the first script but not with the second script.

If this is the case, it may be that the first script speaks to your subconscious mind more effectively than the second script. The reason for this is that your subconscious mind likes to be reminded of the struggle, which the first script talks about and the second does not. To change, some subconscious minds need to see what they have to work against. In other words, the subconscious mind needs an enemy to fight. There is nothing unusual or strange about this—it is true for about 10 percent of my clients. What you should do is go back to your first script. Use it for a week, then come back to this exact sentence and paragraph.

After you have listened to the first script for another week, ask yourself how things are going now. Are they working again? If so, then continue to use the first script every other night until you reach your goal weight and then once a week to maintain your goal. You can now skip ahead to page 237, where I will talk about other things you can do to support your new lifestyle.

It's not the first script or the second script— it is just that you are seeing no change.

If this is the case, then the first thing we look at is the possibility that you are one of the lucky few who fall asleep so easily and quickly that you practically skip the alpha phase and go right into deeper (theta) sleep. If you are skipping the alpha phase of sleep, then of course the recording is not working, as alpha is the channel to the subconscious mind and the time when the recording will be most effective. If you suspect or know that you are a person who falls asleep quickly and sleeps deeply, then the solution for you is to listen to your recording in the morning. Set your alarm half an hour earlier than you would like to get up. When the alarm sounds, put the recording on, set the snooze button or a second alarm for another half hour, and fall back to sleep, listening to your recording. Why does this work? Because you will have had a full night's rest, you will not be as tired, and your brain is less likely to bypass the alpha state altogether. Therefore, your subconscious mind will have the opportunity to tune in.

Begin the process again, using this approach to listen to the first script for ten days, and then use the second script. Please note that even though the language in the second script talks about preparing for the following day, just know as you rehearse the day that it is referring to the day in front of you instead of the following morning. **There is no need to make a new recording.** Listen every morning for two weeks and see if you notice a difference, then come back to this exact sentence.

Listening in the morning rather than at night is also a good solution for people who are finding that listening at night is just impossible because of family distractions (young kids crawling into bed or calling out to you), partner issues, and so on.

Once you have listened to the first script for a week to ten days and the second script for two weeks, ask yourself how you are doing. Better? See a difference? If so, then listen every other morning until you reach your goal weight and then every week or so for life to maintain your new relationship with food. It's also a good idea to use the non-listening-nights exercise. If you have seen a difference by listening in the morning, you can now skip ahead to page 237 to learn more about what else you can do to support your health and well-being.

Your mind does not have enough to think about.

Believe it or not, another thing that can make changes hard for the subconscious mind is that it does not have enough to think about. If a large focus of your life has been thinking about food, planning meals, and eating and you don't have anything else to feel passionate about, then your subconscious mind is going to want to hang on to food. Why? Because it wants something to do! Our brains like to be active, working, engaged. The simple solution for this is to offer the mind something else to think about. Get a hobby. Find a passion. Think about something you used to like to do as a child—painting, drawing, a physical activity—and start doing it again. Or, if you feel you have never been passionate about anything in your life, think about things you would like to try. It does not need to be an extreme sport—it can be as simple as crossword puzzles or knitting. There is no way to combat the brain's boredom other than to occupy the mind. You have to get busy. This will be particularly helpful if you are an after-dinner snacker.

You have too much to think about.

Of course, in this day and age, many of us have the opposite problem: too much to do. Being stressed and being overextended can work against the medical hypnosis process in a number of ways. First and most obviously, if you are really stressed out, your brain may not be able to take on one iota more of information. It just can't. The mere idea of change is too stressful. Your brain is rejecting the idea of change because, like a computer with too many programs running at one time, it is overloaded and crashing. If you find yourself in this boat, then the first thing that you must do is to find a way to alleviate some of your stress.

The simplest solution to stress is meditation. Don't believe me? Try it for two weeks—five minutes a day, a couple of times a day—and see if you feel a difference. I'll tell you exactly how to do it on page 240.

The other thing that you may need to do to alleviate some of your stress is to become more organized. You need to be organized so that you have time for yourself and can take care of your basic needs, such as sleep, eating three proper meals, and even taking a shower (hot water can help to relax the muscles in the body and offer some stress relief). Caretakers—this includes anyone who takes care of another person in any way, such as doctors, lawyers, brokers, parents, nurses, teachers, and CEOs—are particularly prone to making sure everything and everyone else is well and thriving at the cost of their own health. A few years ago, a doctor specializing in obstetrics and gynecology came to see me. Jessica was in her early forties, was married, and had three kids. She was 30 pounds overweight and knew that the combination of her high-stress job and carrying this extra weight was going to lead to disease if she did not address it. When I looked at her life, I saw that medical hypnosis could help her, but also knew that some behavior modification and meditation would serve her more in the long run.

Jessica was a classic stress eater. She was on the go 24/7—if she didn't need to deliver a baby or perform surgery, then it was her own child who needed care. Her eating habits were horrendous. Most days, she would run to the hospital at four in the morning on an empty stomach, deliver babies, and graze on whatever crap was in the doctors' lounge, which was usually bagels or donuts and coffee. Then she would run to meet with patients at her private practice. At lunch, she might eat a salad or half a sandwich or she might not. By the time Jessica got home, she would be starving. She would gorge on whatever was in the house, eating pizza with the kids and then some roast chicken with her husband. Jessica and I talked about what she could do to take better care of herself, and we came up with the solution that she would always have a "go cooler" ready and stocked. This cooler would have healthy food that she could eat when days were particularly stressful. She would prepare several of these coolers for herself on Sundays to ensure that she would have lean protein and vegetables that would nourish her body as she ran through her days. The other thing that we talked about was the idea that Jessica needed to give herself at least two moments of peace during the day. I taught Jessica how to meditate and she began to practice mini meditations throughout her day—anytime there was a moment at the hospital or between clients. These two techniques helped Jessica lose the 30 pounds in no time; more importantly, she found she had more energy and strength to negotiate her challenging days.

Troubleshooting: Phase II

If none of the last four approaches has helped you and you are still struggling, let's keep going. I am not giving up on you yet. So don't give up on yourself.

If little or nothing is happening, the next thing to look at is what psychological issues or emotional pulls might make it too hard for you to lose weight. In particular cases, old messages such as the ones we explored in the "Place Settings" chapter might be so powerful that they cannot be dislodged with a simple release and the proper use of the two scripts. They need to be talked out, addressed, and understood with the help of a therapist before they can be let go. Then there are other clients who have a singular problem they were not aware of until they began the medical hypnosis process, found resistance, and looked more closely at their struggle. If you have a powerful neuropathway for unhealthy eating lodged deep in your brain, it can take a tremendous amount of effort to find it and address it.

About a year ago, a woman named Tanya came to me and told me that her greatest dream was to be thin on her wedding day. She was 40 pounds overweight, but we had a year before her wedding, so I believed her dream was possible. We did the first and second sessions. She listened correctly and yet saw no results.

When she came in for a third session, I suspected we had been focusing on the wrong subject. In the first session, while doing her Inventory, Tanya had told me about how her mother had force-fed her, plied her with sweet snacks, and taught her to use food as a way of comforting herself. But we'd never talked about her relationship with her fiancé. In the third session, we finally did.

Tanya told me that she and John had been together off and on since high school. That he was her "rock." That he was "amazing and the fittest man on the planet." I asked her what she meant by this. She told me that John was a workout addict. He would go to the gym before and after work every day. I asked her how he felt about her body. She told me that he was always bugging her to come to the gym with him and that she sometimes went, but that she appreciated his support and the fact that he was trying to help her with her weight struggle. I said, "Really?" I asked her how long they had been engaged. Without thinking, she said, "Which time?" When I asked her what had happened to the first engagement, Tanya burst into tears and told me that eighteen months earlier, John had left her for a trainer at the gym. Over the years he had left Tanya for a thin woman three times, but he had always come back because he said he really loved Tanya. Of course, reading this story, it is easy to see that John has some major issues and that Tanya shouldn't have been marrying him. As it turned out, that's exactly what her subconscious mind was thinking as well. Her subconscious mind was relying on the fact that if Tanya kept the weight on, John would leave again. Her subconscious mind was protecting her, keeping her from getting too close to something that had caused her deep pain in the past.

I suggested to Tanya that she see a therapist about her relationship with John and that I suspected that her engagement to a man with whom she had such a complicated and painful relationship might be what was really holding her back. These days, she is still seeing the therapist, but not John. And she is finally losing the weight.

As you can see in this story and in others we've talked about throughout the book, weight is often not the issue. Weight can come off and on, but it is the emotional issues that stick to our guts, and it takes perseverance and strength to weed these deep and painful patterns out. I believe, from personal and professional experience, that it is best not to do this alone. You need someone else's ears, perspective, and strength of heart to help you through the process.

Whether you choose to do the looking alone or with a professional, spend the next week or so observing your behavior and the emotions around that behavior. Whom were you with or not with? What were you doing? Where were you? For instance, look at your Life Log and make the connection between the phone call from your best friend and eating a cookie. Or notice that your stress level rises when your kids scream. How are you handling that stress? By yelling back? By eating?

See what comes up, whether you notice anything new about yourself. You should also ask yourself if there is, as with Tanya, a secondary benefit to carrying excess weight. You may have an epiphany. If after a week you have had a revelation about a certain food-behavior-person relationship, think about how you might do a release for this. Do the release, and then try using the first and second scripts as prescribed. You may find that you have cracked your own case.

If after a week or so you are still stumped and still want to make a change, please talk to someone. It cannot hurt. And it can help more than you can imagine.

If you have tried anything and everything and you are still struggling, you may in fact have a medical reason for your weight.

This applies only to the tiniest percentage of my clients, but in my twenty-five years of practice I have always seen a few people each year who need the help of a medical doctor. Get a full blood workup. Have your doctor look for diabetes and thyroid imbalances. These diseases override the entire subconscious/conscious mind system and can be detrimental to your health. So if you have even the smallest suspicion that your body might be systemically out of whack, then please do not delay. See a doctor immediately. If you are morbidly obese, ask your medical doctor about Prader-Willi syndrome, a brain (hypothalamus) abnormality that can cause "bottomless pit" eating. It's pretty rare, but it's a possibility.

Extending Your Health and Well-Being

For those of you who are doing well or finding your way with the medical hypnosis process, the key to continued success is to be vigilant and true to yourself.

Many people who feel a profound difference in their relationship with food will find that, a few weeks into this process, they feel like a hero and stop listening. They think, "I'm fixed. I don't need it anymore." But here is what you need to understand: **The first and second scripts do not erase the old relationship with food.**

When you are listening to your recording, you are laying a new picture over the old pattern. It is like tossing a beautiful throw over an old couch. You need to straighten the throw every few days or the old couch will start to peek through. I promise you, if you stop listening, the old habits and behaviors will come back. If you toss the tape away, you will be throwing yourself and all the work that you have done into the trash.

Keep listening to the second recording (or first, if that worked better for you) every other night until you have reached your goal weight.

If it's easier to do it every night or in the morning, do that. If you like doing the non-listening-nights exercise (see page 229) every other night or morning, then do that too. The point here is to keep doing what you have found works for your own particular subconscious mind.

When you think about what your goal weight is, don't have a number or size in mind. Have a picture of how you want to feel in your body. See yourself as lean, strong, and healthy—empowered. And once you reach that goal, don't try to stay at a specific weight or size. The body's weight naturally fluctuates between three and five pounds—this is particularly true for women.

Likewise, while losing the weight, don't aim for a particular number of pounds per week that you should lose. I have had clients who have lost up to 50 pounds in the first month, but this is unusual. Most lose at a rate of about 2 to 3 pounds a week. Like everything else in life, losing weight is a process. More important than the speed of losing weight is the fact that changing your relationship with food means having new preferences and desires. When good, healthy food is the preference, the weight-loss process is a one-way street: down.

You should know, however that the closer you get to your goal weight, the more slowly you will lose. For instance, a person who weighs 300 pounds and is 150 pounds overweight might be able to lose 10 pounds a week for several weeks because 10 pounds in relationship to his or her starting weight is not that significant. But a person who weighs 140 and is 10 to 15 pounds overweight should not and most likely will not lose 10 pounds in a week—it would be too stressful on the body, and the body knows this. Don't compare yourself to others. Just let the process take its course. Forget the scale and go by how you feel in your clothes and your own skin.

Once you reach your goal weight, be sure to listen once every week or two for the rest of your life. Drawing this new blueprint is never fixed or done. It takes some maintenance. We are all works in progress! The recording operates the same way blood pressure medication works. As long as you take the medicine, your blood pressure will remain steady and under control. This does not mean that if you stop listening to the CD you will immediately go on a binge, but you may notice, depending on the strength of the old patterning, that a few old habits will begin to crop up and you will have less resistance and indifference to these foods and behaviors, and eventually the old pattern will emerge. Think about it. What is going to win, a ten-, twenty-, or thirty-year-old habit or something that is months or a year old?

Milton and Nancy were a married couple who managed a very successful real estate business together. The toll of sharing both a relationship and business was that they were both about 60 pounds overweight. Although they came in for separate appointments, both said that eating was their way of bonding and blowing off the steam and stress of working and living with a partner. After a long day where they had little or nothing to eat, they liked to go to restaurants where there were buffet tables or where the portions were large. There they would, in Nancy's words, "eat like there was no tomorrow."

With both Nancy and Milton, I went through the first and second scripts. They responded beautifully. Both began to feel more in control immediately. They couldn't believe it. Milton was particularly affected by the experience and came to me asking for a method to combat the daily stress of his job. I taught him how to meditate and induce Dr. Benson's Relaxation Response. He was diligent about listening to the recordings, using his Anchor Statement, and meditating. He lost the 60 pounds without thinking twice.

Nancy also did well—that is, until she stopped listening to her recording. When she had about 15 more pounds to lose, she decided that she didn't need the recording or Anchor Statement anymore. She rationalized this decision by thinking that her husband was just weaker and therefore needed to rely on the recording and other steps. She, on the other hand, was strong. Within a month, however, all the old behaviors came back. And in four months, all the weight came back as well.

Nancy felt awful. How had her husband succeeded where she had failed? She came back to me, feeling humiliated and ashamed. I told her that the only way in which she had failed was by not believing that she still needed help. All she needed to do to get back on track was to follow the process through once more. It had worked the first time; she had just stopped using it! So Nancy did the first and second sessions again, and once more she responded beautifully. This time she listened, meditated, and used her Anchor Statement. This time she lost the weight and kept it off.

The moral of this story? Tune in. And be honest with yourself. If you find yourself less inclined to listen to your CD after a few weeks and think you have cracked your case, know that you are only fooling yourself. Of course, even though I have said this and told you this story, in my experience about a third of my clients test this and stop listening. And, unfortunately, that third will, like Nancy, eventually find themselves face-to-face with their old patterns and weight once more.

What if this practice does not resolve every food item?

If you have found that you have seen an 80 percent or greater difference in your food habits and behaviors, then I think you have had a tremendous success. Some people completely and totally resolve every food issue with medical hypnosis. Others find that there are a few sticking points. It may be that these issues just need more time to be kicked out. Or it may be that these foods or behaviors have significant emotional ties that need to be addressed with a therapist before they are let go. If you do have one small habit that is nagging you and not detrimental, it is nothing to fret over. You have made massive changes in your life and you should not worry that you have failed or that this will hold you back. Give it time. Healthy behavior builds and snowballs: Healthy habits and an improved sense of self typically generate a desire to do more healthy, self-empowering things for ourselves.

Meditation: The Ultimate Drug-Free Stress Reliever

If you don't manage stress, it will manage you. Beyond continuing to listen to your recording, the other thing that I strongly recommend to all my clients is to practice meditation. As I said in Chapter 3, meditation is not a religion, nor do you have to give up your religion to practice meditation. It is the simple and direct practice of watching your breath, which slows your heart rate, lowers the body's stress hormones, and increases your sense of well-being and resilience.

The reason it is so important to combat stress is that stress is the number-one reason why any and every overeater eats. Over the years, I have found that life stress—death, job loss, moving, divorce, illness, surgery (particularly involving anesthesia), starting or finishing school or a big project, becoming parents, having a bad boss or coworker, long hours, even ten loads of laundry—can trigger old behaviors to resurface. I know that when I am stressed, the first thing that occurs to me is peanut butter. These days, I know that peanut butter is not going to alleviate my stress (in fact, it will add to it), but in the old days I didn't. Fortunately, because I still listen to my recording and practice meditation, my first response is not "Where's the jar?" but "I wonder what has me so stressed out."

Along with a sense of peace, meditation offers a kind of awareness that serves as a sort of safeguard against old patterns. When a change in our life happens and the wind gets knocked out of us, we always resort to our primal patterning. No drug or therapy or even medical hypnosis is going to change this. But what we can address and work on is our reaction. We may have the thought of food (as I do with peanut butter when I'm stressed), but meditation puts a pause between the thought and the action.

Because you are taking time out for yourself each day to tune in and check up, you will be more aware of what you are doing and better able to identify stressors, understand your emotional triggers, and recognize when you are too busy or bored. Essentially, the practice of meditation is like an emotional thermometer or gauge that tells you what your temperature is. It is a lens for understanding yourself and your relationship with people, places, and things.

There are hundreds if not thousands of ways to practice meditation, and if you are curious, you can go to your local library or bookstore to learn about all the options you have in this department, but the kind of meditation that I practice and have found most effective for addressing stress and promoting health is very simple: **Watch your breath**.

Watching Your Breath

I use this method because it can be done anywhere, anytime. Depending on your needs, desires, and life, you may find that it is easier to practice this method in short spurts of five minutes or in one longer twenty-minute session. I strongly recommend the five-minute version for everyone to begin with, as it is a great way to learn and experience the benefits of meditation without much commitment. I also suggest that if you go with the 5-minute approach, you use this technique several times throughout the day to help moderate and relieve the intensity of your life. You can do it in the bathroom at work, at your desk, on your lunch break, in a hallway, at the doctor's office, waiting to pick up the kids at school, or when you have a craving or feel like snacking. A mini meditation is the best gauge for distinguishing real hunger from cravings. The longer version is for those of you who have found that you like meditating and want more. This twenty-minute version is a truly wonderful way to begin or end a day.

With the five-minute version, the focus is on using the breath to slow the heart rate and drop the blood pressure by picturing ourselves in a relaxing place, which triggers Dr. Benson's Relaxation Response, which I talked about in Chapter 1. This is why I prescribe the five-minute version for people who have high-stress jobs. It offers instant relief, relaxing the muscles, lowering blood pressure, and lowering stress hormone levels.

While the twenty-minute version also uses the breath as a way of relaxing and offers the same physical benefits, the focus is on noticing the breath move in and out of the body rather than picturing ourselves in a relaxing place. Too often, we will watch the breath move in and out for thirty seconds and then suddenly find that our brain has jumped to the day's errands that need to get done, or the dress we want to buy, or our retirement, which is fifteen years away. The twenty-minute meditation is the practice of watching what we think about *without judgment*. Over time, we get to know ourselves better. We learn what we think about during weeks of particular stress—food, shopping, sex— and what we think about when are feeling blue. This is powerful information, offering us a deeper look at who we are and how we move through the world. When we watch our thoughts without judgment, we have the opportunity to watch our reaction—rage, hurt, the desire to stuff ourselves with food—and not immediately engage in the drama. This ability to not live in a state of reaction is what I believe to be true freedom.

Watching your breath: five-minute version

To practice the five-minute version, follow these ten easy steps:

1. Get in a comfortable position (sitting or reclining). If you are sitting up, make sure your feet are supported and resting on the ground and that your arms are resting comfortably on the arms of your chair or in your lap.

2. Close your eyes and take six or seven deep breaths in through your nose and out through your mouth. Then just breathe normally through your nose.

3. Focus on the air coming in and out of your nose. Say your Anchor Statement in your inner voice a few times.

4. Continue to breathe normally and relax all the muscles in your face.

5. Let your head feel heavy (if reclined) so there's no strain in your neck.

6. Let your shoulders and arms feel heavy.

7. Relax your stomach muscles.

8. Let your legs feel heavy. Think of yourself as being as relaxed as a rag doll.

9. To relax even further, picture yourself in the most beautiful place you can imagine. Picture the colors, the smells. The temperature is perfect. Imagine yourself doing something you love to do. Maybe it is lying on a beach in the sun, or reading in the shade under a tree, or playing with your children or grandchildren. Stay in this perfect place where nothing is wrong or can

go wrong. The longer you stay in this place, the more relaxed you'll feel. Stay for at least five minutes, or as long as you like. Toward the end, reinforce your Anchor Statement by repeating it.

10. When you are ready and feel more relaxed, take a deep breath, bringing your attention back to the sounds around you. Stretch your arms and legs. Slowly open your eyes. Take a few more deep breaths to clear your head and bring oxygen to your body. Take your time bringing your attention back to the activity at hand.

Watching your breath: twenty-minute version

Once you've mastered the five-minute version (or just feel comfortable with it), try the twenty-minute version by following these ten easy steps:

1. Get in a comfortable position (sitting or reclining). If you are sitting up, make sure your feet are supported and resting on the ground and that your arms are resting comfortably on the arms of your chair or in your lap.

2. Close your eyes and take eight to ten deep breaths in through your nose and out through your mouth. Then just breathe normally through your nose.

3. Focus on the air coming in and out of your nose. Say your Anchor Statement in your inner voice a few times.

4. Continue to breathe normally and relax all the muscles in your face.

5. Let your head feel heavy (if reclined) so there's no strain in your neck.

6. Let your shoulders and arms feel heavy.

7. Relax your stomach muscles.

8. Let your legs feel heavy. Think of yourself as being as relaxed as a rag doll.

9. Now, just let your breath go. Don't force your breathing. Just let your natural breath move in and out of you. Watch your breath. Notice how it is cooler on the inhale and warmer on the exhale. Focus on the rhythm of your breathing. If your mind drifts, simply notice where it drifted to and bring your focus back to the breath. Continue to do this for twenty minutes. Know that you will lose your breath and find it again many times. This is the practice.

10. When you are ready and feel more relaxed, take a deep breath, bringing your attention to the sounds around you. Stretch your arms and legs. Slowly open your eyes. Take a few more deep breaths to clear your head and bring oxygen to your body. Take your time bringing your attention back to the activity at hand.

As with everything, the practice of meditation takes time to get used to, so please give it and yourself a chance. Don't do it once and say, "It's not for me." Try doing at least one mini meditation for seven days and see if you feel a difference. Know that there is no right or wrong way to meditate. If you lose track of your breath, don't worry about it. This is completely natural. It is just your brain trying to speed itself up, which, as you well know, it loves to do. Smile at your silly mind, then go back to your breath and ease back into the idea of the meditation at hand.

Our Last Supper

For the last few weeks I have been meditating and thinking about what words of advice and thoughts I want to leave you with. In one meditation, I had this wonderful fantasy that I would suddenly write something, like a new version of the Ten Commandments, that was so brilliant and fantastic that every reader would read it and then have an epiphany and never struggle with food ever again. I don't like to be "commanded" any more than the next person, but this fantasy was motivated by my truest and most honest desire: that people stop struggling with their weight. So I leave you with my ten best thoughts:

1. May you be lean, strong, and healthy.

2. May you support your health and well-being by listening to your recording and to yourself.

3. May you expand your mind. Be curious about your outer and inner life. Meditate.

4. As I've said, retraining your brain and learning to value yourself and your body take time. Give yourself this time.

5. Value yourself. Your life is as precious as a newborn's. Treat yourself accordingly.

6. Try new things. As your body shrinks, your world will expand. Be fearless.

7. Listen to your body. If you are tired, sleep. If you are truly hungry, eat. If you are full, don't eat.

8. No matter how much you hate it, move your body. Your heart will love you for it. And your grandchildren will be glad they got to meet and know you.

9. May you have love in your life—friends, family, partners. There's nothing else like it.

10. May you laugh at yourself or with others at least once a day. Life just isn't that serious, even when we're challenging ourselves.

I hope that by now you have learned that there is so much more to life than eating. So embrace it. We only live once.

This is the end.

And your beginning.

May you be lean, strong, healthy, happy, and free. And may your inner voice be the loudest and strongest of all.

Works Cited

Chapter One: Thin Is a State of Mind

1. http://www.cdc.gov/nchs/fastats/overwt.htm.

2. www.cdc.gov/PDF/Frequently_Asked_Questions_About_Calculating_Obesity-Related_Risk.pdf.

3. S. J. Olshansky, D. J. Passaro, R. C. Hershow, J. Layden, B. A. Carnes, J. Brody, L. Hayflick, R. N. Butler, D. B. Allison, and D. S. Ludwig, "A Potential Decline in Life Expectancy in the United States in the 21st Century," *New England Journal of Medicine,* March 17, 2005, 352:11, pp. 1138–45.

4. http://jama.ama-assn.org/cgi/content/full/295/1/27?maxtoshow_&HIT . . . +level+recommendations&searchid=1&FIRSTINDEX=0&resource-type+HWCIT.

5. http://www.obesity.org/subs/fastfacts/Obesity_Consumer_Protect.shtml.

6. http://www.starbucks.com/retail/nutrition_beverage_detail.asp.

7. http://www.cfsan.fda.gov/~dms/wgtloss.html.

8. http://www.obesity.org/subs/fastfacts/Obesity_Consumer_Protect.shtml.

9. Testimony of Herbert Benson, M.D., "Mind/Body Interventions, Healthcare and Mind/Body Medical Centers," before the United States Senate Appropriations Subcommittee on Labor/HHS and Education, Senator Arlen Specter, Chairman, September 22, 1998.

10. Ibid.

11. http://www.n-shap-ericksonian.co.uk/Erickson.htm.

12. www.nyseph.org/whathypnosis.html.

13. http://www.hersheys.com/products/details/hersheysbar.asp.

14. http://www.leancuisine.com/Products/NutritionInformation.aspx?ProductID=10606.

Chapter Three: The Alpha Solution

1. www.calorie-count.com/calories/item/83655.html.

2. http://www.dunkindonuts.com/aboutus/nutrition/Product.aspx?Category=Beverages&id=DD-959.

3. David Bjerklie, Alice Park, Davide Van Biema, Karen Ann Cullotta, and Jeanne McDowell, "The Science of Meditation," *Time,* August 4, 2003, pp. 49–56.

4. Herbert Spiegel and David Spiegel, *Trance and Treatment: Clinical Uses of Hypnosis,* American Psychiatric Publishing, Arlington, VA, 2nd edition (April 30, 2004), p. 17.

5. http://www.nhlbi.nih.gov/health/public/heart/obesity/lose_wt/recommen.htm.

Chapter Four: Change Your Mind, Change Your Body

1. Arran Frood, *The Photographic Atlas of the Body,* Firefly Books Ltd., New York, 2004, p. 188.

2. Daniel G. Amen, *Change Your Brain, Change Your Life,* Three Rivers Press, New York, 1998, p. 37.

3. Ibid., pp. 38–42.

4. Ibid.

5. Ibid., p. 82.

6. Jeffrey M. Schwartz and Sharon Begley, *The Mind and the Brain,* Regan Books, New York, 2002, p. 68.

7. Amen, *Change Your Brain, Change Your Life,* pp. 82–96.

8. Schwartz and Begley, *The Mind and the Brain,* p. 67.

9. John Ratey, ed., *The Neuropsychiatry of Personality Disorders,* Blackwell Science, Cambridge, Mass., 1995, p. 153.

10. Amen, *Change Your Brain, Change Your Life,* pp. 150–53.

11. Ibid., pp. 186–91.

12. Schwartz and Begley, *The Mind and the Brain,* p. 15.

13. Ibid., p. 101.

14. Ibid., p. 111.

15. S. W. Lazar, C. Kerr, R. H. Wasserman, J. R. Gray, D. Greve, M. T. Treadway, M. McGarvey, B. T. Quinn, J. A. Dusek, H. Benson, S. L. Rauch, C. I. Moore, and B. Fischl, "Meditation Experience Is Associated with Increased Cortical Thickness," *NeuroReport,* 2005;16:1893–97.

Chapter Five: Place Settings

1. www.nhlbi.nih.gov/health/public/heart/obesity/wecan/learn-it/index.htm.

About the Author

Ronald J. Glassman, Ph.D., M.P.H., was educated at Rutgers, Columbia, and the world-renowned Harvard Medical School Mind-Body Institute. He is board-certified in medical hypnosis, neurolinguistic programming (NLP), and sports and performance enhancement and is director and founder of the Ivy League Clinical Hypnosis Center in Manhattan and Mountainside, New Jersey. He has more than twenty-five years of health care experience.

A member in good standing of numerous professional organizations, he was named 2005 Researcher of the Year by The International Association of Counselors and Therapists for his work in understanding the subconscious mind. In 2002, that same organization nominated him for Educator of the Year in recognition of his patient education skills.

An adjunct professor of sociology, philosophy, and psychology, he has also guest lectured and presented at grand rounds at medical schools and hospitals around the country, among them New York University School of Medicine, Columbia University College of Physicians and Surgeons, Robert Wood Johnson Medical School, as well as at Harvard-affiliated hospitals. Dr. Glassman has been conducting original research since 1981. He is currently a Visiting Scientist and Guest Lecturer at Columbia University's Functional Magnetic Resonance Imaging Center.

As a community service, Dr. and Mrs. Glassman underwrite workshops on stress management for individuals undergoing cancer treatment.

Born and raised in Passaic, New Jersey, by his mom, Shirley, a registered nurse, and dad, Paul, a factory worker and photographer, Dr. Glassman resides with his wife, Meryl, in Mountainside, New Jersey.

Mollie Doyle is a freelance writer who lives in Sag Harbor, New York. Her latest projects include *The Alpha Solution* and *A Memory, a Monologue, a Rant, and a Prayer*, writings on violence against women and girls, which she co-edited with Eve Ensler.